11-2-99

Every Bride Is
Beautiful

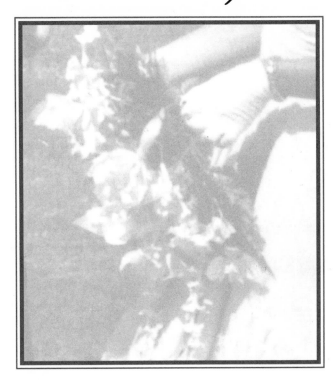

Also by Deborah Chase

Terms of Adornment

Fruit Acids for Fabulous Skin

The New Medically Based No-Nonsense Beauty Book

Dying at Home with Hospice

Extend-Your-Life Diet

The Medically Based No-Nonsense Beauty Book

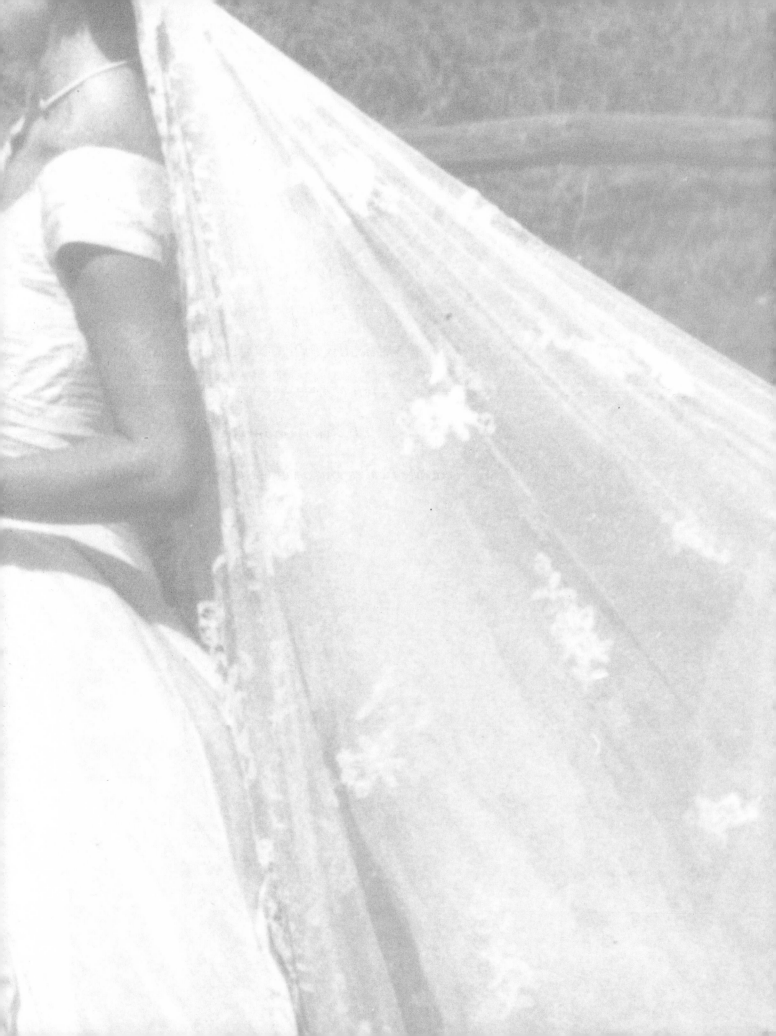

Every Bride Is Beautiful

THE COMPLETE GUIDE TO WEDDING BEAUTY FROM HEAD TO TOE

Deborah Chase

WILLIAM MORROW AND COMPANY, INC.
NEW YORK

Copyright © 1999 by Deborah Chase

It is the policy of William Morrow and Company, Inc., and its imprints and affiliates,
recognizing the importance of preserving what has been written, to print the books we publish
on acid-free paper, and we exert our best efforts to that end.

LIBRARY OF CONGRESS CATALOGING-IN-PUBLICATION DATA
Chase, Deborah.
    Every Bride Is Beautiful: The complete guide to wedding beauty from head to toe/
Deborah Chase.
        p.   cm.
    ISBN 0-688-15426-3
    1. Weddings—United States—planning.   2. Beauty, Personal—United States.   3. Wedding
costume—United States.   I. Title.
HQ745.C43 1999
395.2'2—dc21   98-30163
                                                                                                      CIP

Printed in the United States of America

First Edition

1 2 3 4 5 6 7 8 9 10

BOOK DESIGN BY BTDnyc

www.williammorrow.com

To my husband, Neil,

who after all these years still calls me

his "beautiful bride"; and

to my daughters, Karen and Lauren Schachter,

who cheerfully endured hours of hair and makeup experiments

to road test beauty techniques for this book

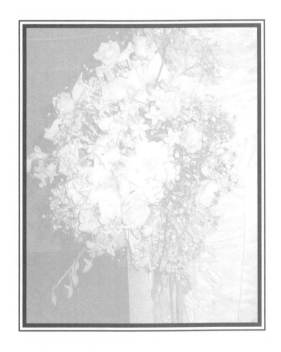

Contents

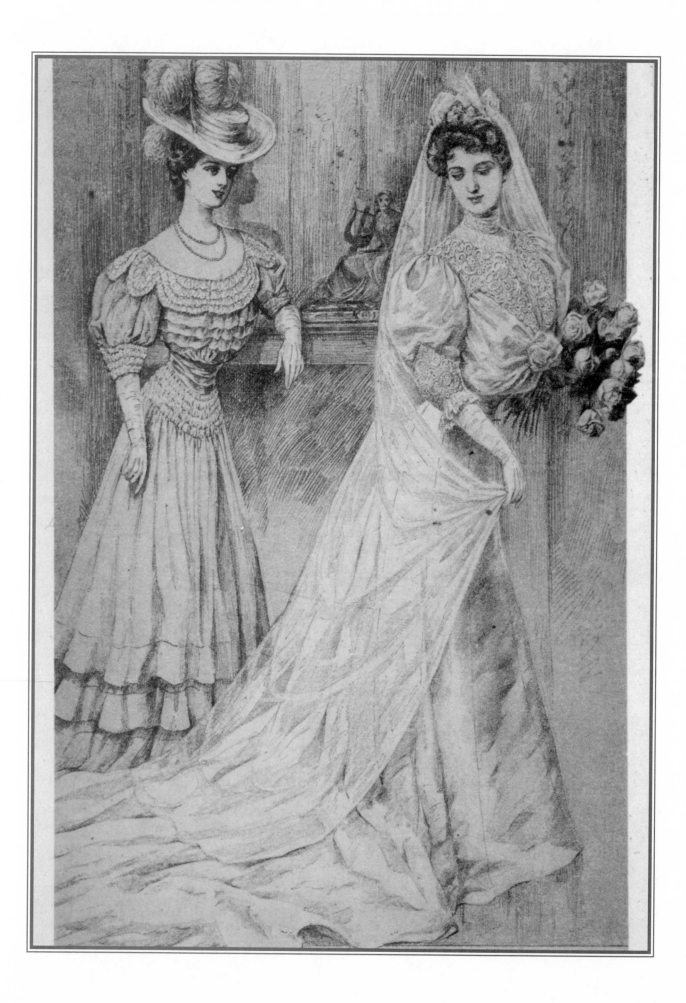

Acknowledgments

One of the great joys of being a writer is the chance to meet new and interesting people, talented men and women who selflessly share their experience and knowledge. I would like especially to thank Marcy Blum, an extraordinary wedding planner with an unfailing sense of bridal styles and organization (as well as a contagious sense of humor); Doris Cooper, a loyal editor whose skill and insight sharpened the focus of the book; Laura Geller, the celebrated makeup artist who opened the doors of her salon to show me what it takes to be a beautiful bride; Monica Hickey, elegant director of custom couture at the bridal salon at Saks Fifth Avenue, whose style and taste helped me understand the dynamics of the flawless wedding ensemble; Chuck Jones of Elizabeth Arden, the hair stylist whose skill and sense of style literally defines the contemporary up-do and who allowed me the opportunity to watch a master work; Rachel Leonard, fashion director of *Bride's* magazine, who combines a modern sensibility with traditional wedding etiquette, offering invaluable insight into personal bridal style; Celle Lalli, longtime editor in chief of *Modern Bride*, whose approach to bridal beauty helped shaped the focus of my chapters on diet and exercise; Stacy Marrison, editor in chief of *Modern Bride,* who generously shared beautiful photographs for the book's cover; Denise O'Donoghue, beauty editor of *Bride's* magazine, whose suggestions and advice were always absolutely perfect. And last, but never least, my agent, Al Zuckerman, of Writer's House, whose singular sense of the publishing market helped reshape my approach to this book as well as my career.

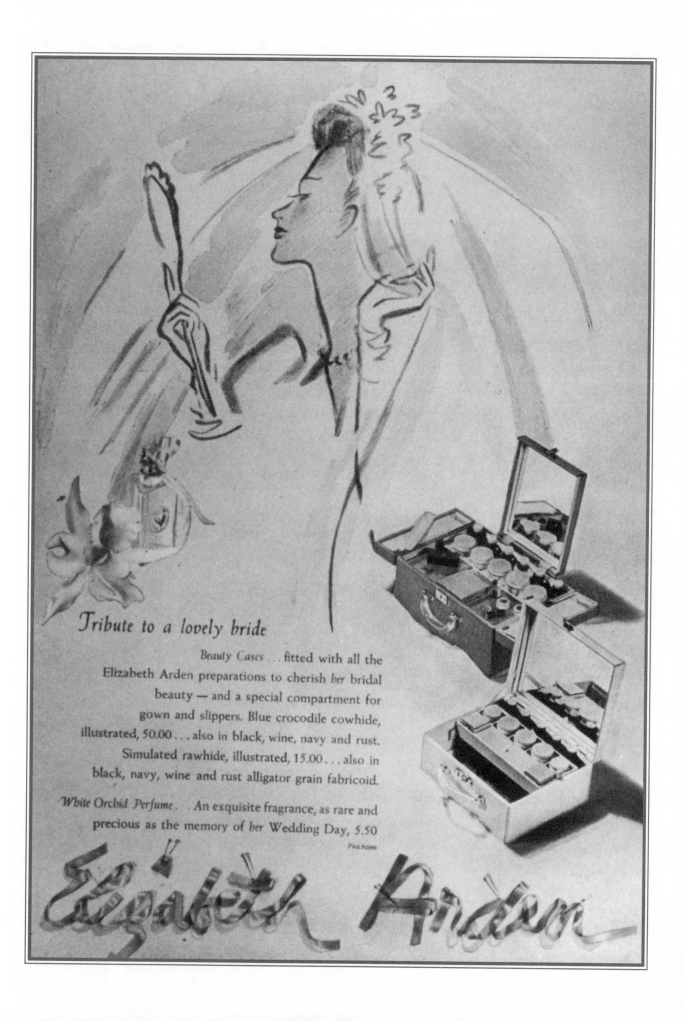

Tribute to a lovely bride

Beauty Cases...fitted with all the
Elizabeth Arden preparations to cherish *her* bridal
beauty — and a special compartment for
gown and slippers. Blue crocodile cowhide,
illustrated, 50.00...also in black, wine, navy and rust.
Simulated rawhide, illustrated, 15.00...also in
black, navy, wine and rust alligator grain fabricoid.

White Orchid Perfume...An exquisite fragrance, as rare and
precious as the memory of *her* Wedding Day, 5.50

Elizabeth Arden

Introduction

Andrea had dreamed and planned for her wedding day since she was a child. At six, she insisted on wearing her "Tiny Tot" wedding dress on the first day of school. At fourteen, she sent away for all the catalogs offered in a bridal magazine, flooding her mailbox with wedding advertisements for more than a year. But when her boyfriend asked her to marry him in a July ceremony, the first thing that occurred to Andrea was her hair. "Heat and humidity turns my thick, curly hair into a frizzy, shapeless mass," she admitted ruefully. "I know it sounds so trivial, but the thought of walking down the aisle with 'July hair' was too awful to contemplate."

Halfway across the country, Dawn was a December bride who hated the idea of makeup, much to the dismay of her mother and aunts. "Foundation feels greasy and suffocating, and eyeliner makes my eyes tear. But everyone is telling me that I'll look terrible in the wedding photographs," she complained.

Midwestern bride-to-be Caroline had no problem with her makeup and her straight, shoulder-length hair offered a smorgasbord of wedding style choices. But her eyeglasses, which she had worn since the fifth grade, clearly presented a challenge. She did not like contacts and did not want to take off her glasses. "I don't want to grope my way blindly through the wedding, but every headpiece looks cluttered and frumpy when worn with my glasses," she explained.

Andrea, Dawn, and Caroline are not unique. Each year more than three million brides are challenged with very specific beauty questions:

* Which headpiece works best for short hair?
* What shade of lipstick photographs best?
* How do you apply makeup that lasts for ten hours?
* Which dress style works for petite silhouettes?

The logistics of a wedding presents hair and fashion issues need to be mastered in the months before a ceremony; but this is not the time for trial and error.

Bridal Learning Curve

Personal style develops over time. We learn which colors work for us, and what styles add five pounds around the hips. With wedding beauty and fashion needs, we do not have the time for mistakes. By the time a bride realizes that her hair needs a little height at the crown to balance her fingertip-length veil or that a matte foundation would have worked better for photographs, the wedding is over. *Every Bride Is Beautiful* will provide essential information when it is needed in the months before the wedding.

For Andrea, it will explain how to use creme rinse and a hot air brush to relax curly hair in humid weather; for Dawn, *Every Bride Is Beautiful* will suggest a rosy moisturizer that will provide sheer light color on the face; for Caroline, it will recommend a smooth, sleek hairstyle and a veil worn without a headpiece. *Every Bride Is Beautiful* will help a bride to sort through the different styles of weddings, dresses, hairstyles, fabrics, and headpieces to select the one that best reflects her taste and personality.

It's Not Vanity

Many brides feel somewhat uncomfortable with the pressure to look beautiful, feeling that they have become self-absorbed and vain. Not true. The image of the beautiful bride is as old as the origins of the wedding itself. For centuries, marriages were arranged between families for political alliance and financial gain. When the bride walked down the aisle, she was a visible symbol of a family's wealth and status. Because the future of both families depended on the success of the marriage, the bride was painstakingly groomed and gowned to reflect all that was viewed as valued and beautiful in a woman.

The Medieval Bride

·············

In a time when knights competed in jousts and women created exquisite tapestries, the medieval bride wore a beautiful dress in brilliant jewel colors. On her head she placed a wreath of flowers, symbolizing purity.

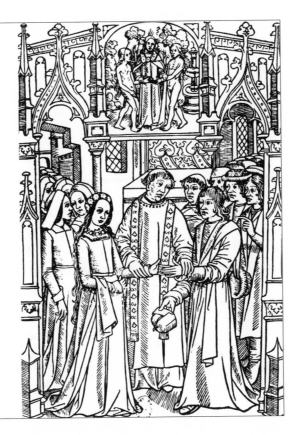

Arranged marriages have disappeared from most cultures, but the intense interest in a bride's appearance has remained. The chapters of *Every Bride Is Beautiful* detail what needs to be done before the wedding as well as tips and techniques on the day of the ceremony. It includes a specially designed diet and exercise program, skin, hair, and nail care plans, the seven wedding makeup styles, and the best bridal hairstyles.

To coordinate beauty plans, *Every Bride Is Beautiful* offers a six-month fitness and beauty calendar. Not only will it provide essential information when it is needed, it establishes a healthy lifestyle program that you can follow in the years to come.

Every Bride Is Beautiful will illustrate many principles of bridal beauty by analyzing the wedding styles of famous brides, including Diana Spencer, Celine Dion, Grace Kelly, Vanessa Williams, Julia Roberts, and Queen Victoria. Their fashion and beauty problems and the solutions they chose offer insight and reassurance for every woman as she prepares to walk down the aisle.

Every Bride Is
Beautiful

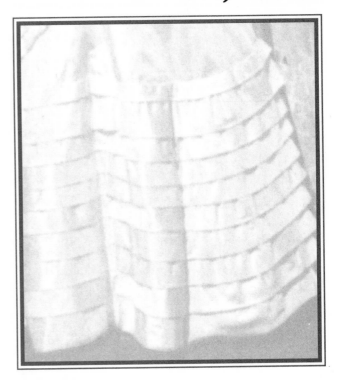

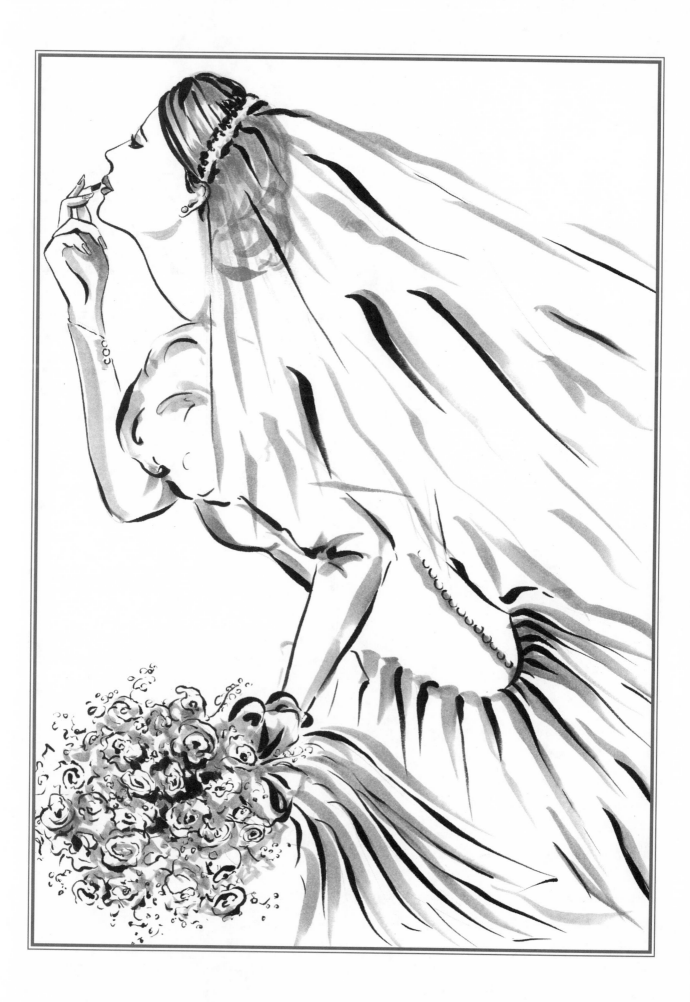

CHAPTER ONE

The Elements of Bridal Style

goals:
....

* **To understand different wedding functions**
* **To determine your personal bridal style**

What kind of dress should I wear? Where will the wedding be held? How should I wear my hair? What kind of makeup should I use? From the moment she gets engaged, a bride has a new question and decision to make each day. It's not trivial or superficial to care about the details of the ceremony and reception. The wedding is a visible symbol of the love and commitment between two people and their desire to share their happiness with friends and family.

It is also an occasion when, for the entire day, the bride is the center of attention. Every eye will be on her, taking in each detail of her appearance. When the wedding is over, the photographs and videos will preserve the wedding image for the rest of her life. It is hardly surprising then that a bride is swamped with details. There seem to be endless choices for every question, but you need not be confused by this. When you start your plans by understanding the etiquette of different wedding ceremonies, as well as your personal bridal style, you will find that the right choices for all your wedding's elements fall naturally into place.

The Origins of Wedding Traditions

Contemporary wedding ceremonies are a tapestry of two thousand years of tradition. They are a blend of royal pageantry, medieval superstitions, Edwardian sentimentality, and the Victorian passion for etiquette.

Etiquette began in the court of Louis XIV. The king's gardener, angry

The Renaissance Bride

············

The sixteenth-century bride wore an elegant and jeweled gown in any color except green, which was thought to bring bad luck. To conform with Renaissance beauty standards, she would pluck out her eyebrows and pull her hair back tightly to create a high, smooth forehead. In homage to Queen Elizabeth, the Renaissance bride used a white powder on her face, rouge on her cheeks, and red pigment on her lips. To keep her makeup fresh, she would cover her face with a glaze of egg whites.

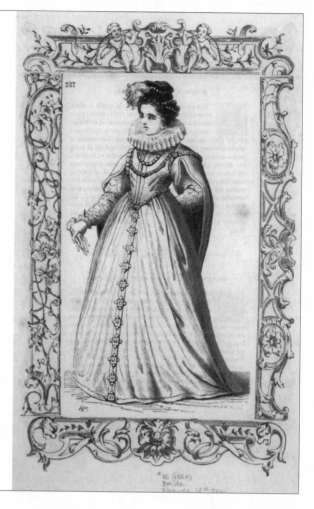

at the crowds that trampled his flower beds, set up signs called "etiquettes" directing where people should walk. When the ladies and gentlemen of the court ignored the signage, the gardener complained to the king. In response, Louis declared that people must observe the "etiquettes." In time, etiquette became the practice of observing courteous, respectful behavior that made life comfortable for all citizens.

Over the centuries, etiquette traditions were established by kings and queens and followed without question by their subjects. As the Industrial Revolution created new wealth and an increasingly prosperous middle class, etiquette became the rules by which respectable people conducted both private lives and public celebrations.

While rules and manners of etiquette existed before the Victorians, no one has ever equaled their enthusiasm for regulating behavior. Each aspect of their lives, from the moment they woke up to the moment they fell asleep, were analyzed and ordered. Each situation had a designated wardrobe, place, date, time, menu, and behavior.

Along with gas lamps and buggy whips, most Victorian etiquette rules have vanished from the social radar; but for wedding etiquette, time has stood still. Our current guidelines for the formality or informality of a wedding were created by Victorians, not to show people what they were doing wrong, but to help the emerging middle class feel comfortable on the most important social event of their lives. Victorian sensibilities have evolved into a quartet of wedding styles that range from small and casual to large and regal.

Grand and elaborate, ultraformal weddings have a guest list of at least 250 friends, family, and acquaintances. They are held either in the afternoon or evening, in a cathedral, a grand synagogue, or an elegant hotel. The bride is accompanied by six to twelve bridesmaids and groomsmen, the bridesmaids all in full-length gowns. It is the only type of wedding where the bridesmaids can wear white. The groom will wear a cutaway for the day and white tie and tails if the wedding is in the evening. The bride's elaborate dress has a train, the longest train that she wishes to wear, and at least a floor-length veil.

After the wedding, there is a full reception, a seated dinner with live music, dancing, champagne, and a multilayered cake. This type of wedding was once reserved for state or royal weddings, such as the wedding of Prince Charles and Lady Diana Spencer. Since the turn of the century, it has been the elaborate wedding choice for very well-known or wealthy couples such as the marriage of singer Celine Dion to Rene Angélil at Notre Dame Basilica in Montreal, Canada. Given the sheer size and grandeur of an ultraformal wedding, the price tag usually starts at $50,000 and can easily run up into the high six figures.

By contrast, the formal wedding, which is announced with engraved cards and envelopes inside envelopes, has between 75 and 250 guests and is held in a mansion, country club, or hotel, as well as a church or synagogue and (unlike the ultraformal wedding, which is held indoors) can take place outdoors in garden settings. The bride is accompanied by three to six bridesmaids in long dresses of any color but white. The groom will wear a

quick tip:

Guide to Groom's Clothing

CUTAWAY: Also known as a morning coat, the long black or gray jacket is traditionally accompanied by gray vest and striped pants. It is worn at formal and ultraformal weddings.

STROLLER: A shorter version of the cutaway, this coat is best for formal or semiformal weddings.

TUXEDO: Also known as black tie, the black peaked jacket and pants trimmed with black satin are worn after 6:00 P.M. for formal and semiformal weddings. From May 15 to September 15, it is appropriate for a groom to wear a white tuxedo jacket with the pants.

WHITE TIE AND TAILS: The black tailcoat paired with a white pique tie and vest is the most elegant choice for ultraformal evening weddings.

Every Bride Is Beautiful

5

stroller for a day wedding and a black or white dinner jacket if the ceremony takes place after 6 P.M.

After the ceremony, the meal can be either a plated dinner or a buffet, but the guests must have assigned seats. The bride's gown can be a full ball gown shape with a chapel or sweep train, which is shorter than the train for the ultraformal wedding. The veil should at least reach the fingertips but can be long enough to just sweep the floor.

The semiformal wedding has between 50 and 150 guests and can be held in a home, hotel, or club. Sometimes it can be a small ceremony followed by a large reception. The choice of reception is expanded to unusual and beautiful sites, such as a yacht, botanical garden, roof of a skyscraper, or country inn. Meal choices can depend on the time of the wedding. Midday weddings can offer tea sandwiches, and afternoon services can be followed by a cocktail buffet, while an evening ceremony can be preceded by cocktails and followed by a dinner.

There are up to three bridesmaids, and they can wear short or long dresses. Men wear the classic dinner jacket in the evening and a suit during the day. The wedding gown should reach the floor or have just a small sweep train. The veil should be no shorter than the shoulders and no longer than fingertip-length.

The semiformal wedding is one of the most popular wedding styles, because it gives the bride the beauty and the formality that we associate with weddings, but at a much more manageable size. It is a favorite wedding style in warm weather climates because of the availability of so many wonderful outdoor resources and a greater chance of good weather.

The informal wedding sends engraved, handwritten, or telephoned invitations to up to fifty guests. The vows can be taken in a hotel suite or home, or the entire wedding party can travel to a special site, like a country inn or yacht. There are no set rules for the reception. It can be as simple as champagne and cake, or it can be a sit-down dinner in a country garden or cocktails on a beach.

The bride can choose to wear a dressy suit, a short or ballerina-length dress, or a long gown if it is a simple, narrow style. There is usually just a single bridesmaid in a dress that matches the length of the bride's clothing. The groom wears a dark suit. This was the wedding style of Carolyn Bessette and John Fitzgerald Kennedy, Jr., demonstrating that the informal wedding can be elegant and beautiful, albeit simple in style and scope. The young couple rented out an old inn on an island off the coast of Georgia to accommodate fifty close friends and family members. The bride wore an off-white, bias-cut charmeuse silk slip dress, while the groom was in a navy suit. They were wed by candlelight in a rustic nineteenth-century church built and used by slaves.

Mixing and Matching

To avoid problems planning a wedding, try to avoid the temptation to mix and match features of all four wedding styles. From a cultural standpoint, we have absorbed the traditions of what looks right or feels right in a wedding, much the way we've absorbed the traditions of Thanksgiving. Even a preschooler anticipates a golden brown turkey, sweet potatoes, and cranberry sauce at Thanksgiving. A Thanksgiving dinner that features steamed lobsters, clams, and roasted corn on the cob will be delicious, but it will somehow not quite feel like Thanksgiving.

The same problems will arise in a wedding if you start mixing and combining features of formality and informality in the same event. If you absolutely feel that you must do a wedding your own way, remember that an informal wedding will provide you the greatest flexibility for your own original choices and style.

Personal Wedding Styles

As you think about what type of wedding you want, you need to identify your personal bridal style. While we are all individuals with our own likes and dislikes, interests and values, brides throughout the United States fall into five distinctive patterns: romantic, traditional, contemporary, California, and European.

In order to have a wedding that best reflects your taste and personality, take this little quiz. As you read through the questions, a pattern will emerge that will help you create a wonderful blend of honored traditions with personal style.

1. **If you are driving with your fiancé and surfing the radio, the song you would stop at would be**
   a. "Because You Loved Me" (Celine Dion)
   b. "When a Man Loves a Woman" (Percy Sledge)
   c. "It Had to Be You" (Harry Connick, Jr.)
   d. "Crazy" (Patsy Cline)
   e. Pachelbel's *Canon*

2. **Your favorite story book when you were a young girl was**
   a. *Cinderella*
   b. *Wuthering Heights* (Charlotte Brontë)
   c. *Where the Sidewalk Ends* (Shel Silverstein)
   d. *A Very Young Skater* (Jill Krementz)
   e. *The Little Prince* (Saint-Exupéry)

3. **Your idea of a perfect vacation would be**
   a. a week in a castle in Scotland
   b. a week in Bermuda
   c. trekking through Nepal
   d. an extreme sports package
   e. a week at the Hôtel du Cap in the South of France

4. **The most romantic form of transportation would be**
   a. horse and carriage
   b. Mercedes SL
   c. Range Rover
   d. Corvette
   e. Bugatti

5. **If money was no object, your choice of a home would be**
   a. a plantation in Georgia
   b. a colonial on Cape Cod
   c. a townhouse in San Francisco
   d. a horse ranch in Montana
   e. a villa in Tuscany

6. **Your ultimate romantic movie is**
   a. *The English Patient*
   b. *Roman Holiday*
   c. *When Harry Met Sally*
   d. *Field of Dreams*
   e. *Like Water for Chocolate*

7. **If you could choose a dream date, it would be**
   a. Cary Grant
   b. Tom Cruise
   c. Nicholas Cage
   d. Pete Sampras
   e. Antonio Banderas

8. **You love the look and style of**
   a. Princess Diana
   b. Jacqueline Kennedy Onassis
   c. Gwyneth Paltrow
   d. Christie Brinkley
   e. Juliette Binoche

9. **Your favorite meal with your fiancé is**
   a. a candlelit dinner
   b. Thanksgiving dinner
   c. a fusion dinner
   d. beach picnic
   e. dinner for two at Tour d'Argent

ANALYSIS OF THE TEST

If you answered mostly A, you are romantic, nostalgic, dreamy, and feminine. You love to dress up and spend a lot of time looking for Mr. Right. You like cuddling kittens, the feel of silk on skin, long, often curly hair, champagne, chocolate, and strawberries. You enjoy chiffon, *Gone With the Wind*, ruffles, and Frank Sinatra. Sometimes called the Princess Bride syndrome, you love the formality of pomp and circumstance, and you tend to dream of the more formal type of wedding. The ultimate romantic bride was Lady Diana Spencer.

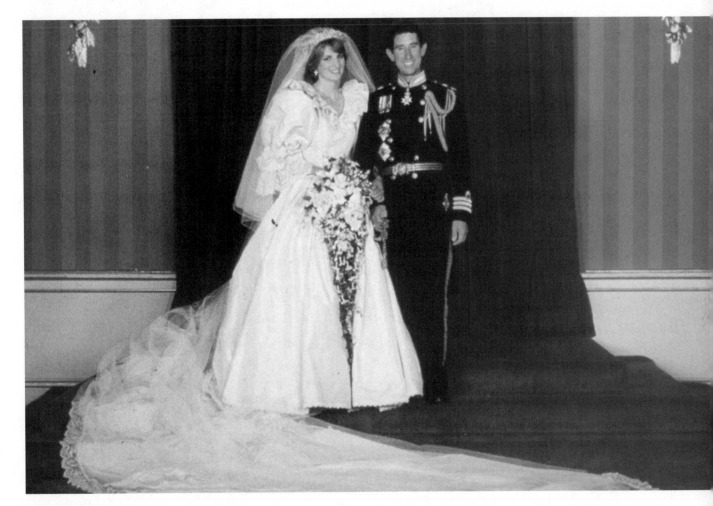

A Romantic Bride

The wedding gown was made with ivory silk taffeta topped with an overlay of pearl-embellished Carrickmacross lace, which had originally belonged to Queen Mary. The frilly large collar, the full puffed elbow-length sleeves, and a twenty-five-foot train were designed to meet the grandeur of St. Paul's Cathedral. A tiny olive bow was stitched into the waistband for good luck. Diana's veil was embroidered with pearls and secured to her head with the two-hundred-year-old diamond Spencer tiara.

Every Bride Is Beautiful

9

Grace Kelly: The Traditional Bride

The bridal dress and veil for the wedding of Grace Kelly and Prince Rainier is considered by many wedding consultants to be a perfect example of a traditional bridal look. The ivory lace gown, with a cathedral train and a delicate, pearl-studded Juliet cap, were created by movie costume designer Helen Rose. Her entire ensemble was intended to be as beautiful on film and in photographs as it was in person at the Grand Palais in Monte Carlo. The small cap and cathedral-length veil were designed to focus attention on the bride's beautiful face. Her hair was swept back in a shining, smooth chignon and accessorized with a pair of simple pearl earrings. Kelly was careful to darken her brows and use a slightly darker shade of lipstick, which would be flattering both on black-and-white TV (there was no color in 1956) and in still photography. Forty years later the effect is as radiant as it was on the day of the wedding.

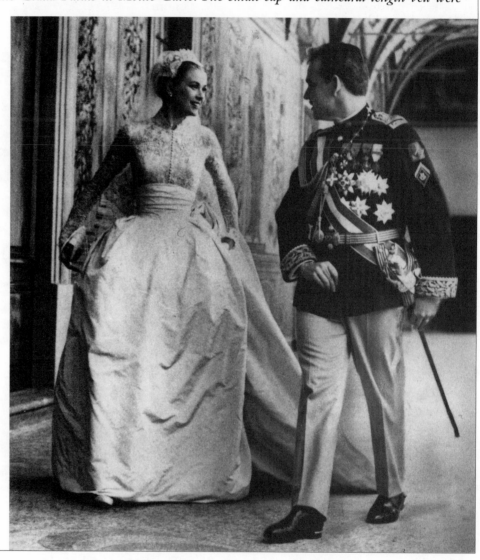

If you answered mostly B, you're a traditional bride. You like classic, timeless clothing—no frills or ruffles. You enjoy wearing good black pumps and a beautiful string of pearls. Your musical choices run from the Beatles to Bach, and you sometimes think you're addicted to decaf skim lattes. You exercise for health rather than fun, and your midlength hair is simple yet polished. You have several pieces of good gold jewelry, rather than a drawerful of lesser items. Your favorite fabrics include cashmere, silk, and velvet, and you would hate to lose your Burberry raincoat. Your tailored and traditional style of a wedding is more formal than informal, but without the clutter. Your gown would be made of luxurious fabrics in simple, classic lines, reminiscent of the wedding dress worn by Grace Kelly.

If you answered mostly Cs, you are a contemporary bride. You own at least six pair of black pants and an equal number of black shoes. Your hair is usually straight, either short or long. You have a toned, slim body, and you don't let a headache or sore throat stop you from your workout. You like Jamba Juice, Elsa Peretti silver jewelry and "indie" movies. You work 24 and 7, and the thought of losing your Filofax makes you shudder. You probably know the fat content of almost any food that finds its way in front of you. The perfect contemporary bridal look is the minimalist elegance of Carolyn Bessette or the lean spare style of Julia Roberts.

The contemporary bride would probably be happiest with a semiformal or informal wedding in which she can express her own chic, simple style in an elegant and original format. Her ideal wedding gown is long and narrow rather than full, and usually devoid of any beading, lace, or trimmings.

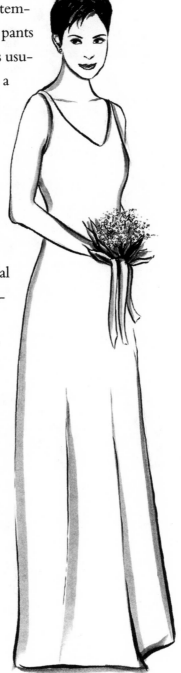

The Contemporary Bride

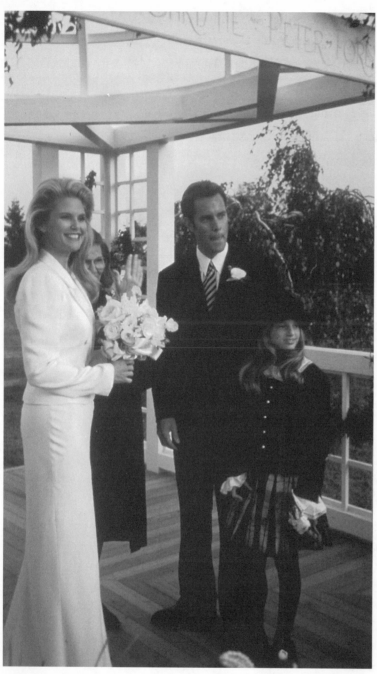

The California
Bride

If you answered mostly D, you are a sunny California, natural, outdoor bride. This is a woman who looks forward to having sons. She loves sports, both watching and participating in them. She may have been on the college team—Varsity. She loves dogs, burgers, fries, and J. Crew sweaters, and she lives in blue jeans. She rarely wears black and often carries a duffel bag or backpack rather than a purse. She likes simple, casual styles that go with her outdoor persona and bright blonde hair. She doesn't like to wear a lot of makeup, and she won't want to wear makeup for the wedding. It is hard to think of this sporty, natural bride in anything but a semiformal or informal wedding that is held in a wonderful outdoor site. The gown would be of soft cotton, organdy, or crepe, rather than stiff tulle or heavy silk. The neckline and sleeves would be styled after street clothes rather than feature traditional bridal details. Christie Brinkley is a perfect example of a California bride.

If you answered mostly E, you're a European bride. You love brocade, fur-trimmed jackets, Manolo Blahnik shoes, and the Concorde. You're probably bilingual and own at least one piece of Versace. You like the look of gold or fur trimming on your bridal dress. The stylings are more fashion-oriented, often with a historical flavor, such as unusual Renaissance sleeves or Victorian necklines. Your wedding makeup is dramatic rather than subtle with smoky eyes and darker lipsticks. Examples of the European bridal style would be the eighteenth-century-inspired dress of Celine Dion.

When a bride identifies the wedding style that best reflects her personality, she will be able to adapt that style to both the makeup and dress silhouette that is most flattering to her face and body. But before she starts to shop for the perfect wedding gown, she needs to evaluate her skin, hair, and shape to make the most of her own natural beauty. If her skin looks dull and blotchy or if her hair is dry and damaged, even the most extraordinary gown will not look its best. The next three chapters will help a bride master skin, dental, and hair care as well as provide a diet and exercise program designed specifically to shape the key areas for a spectacular wedding silhouette.

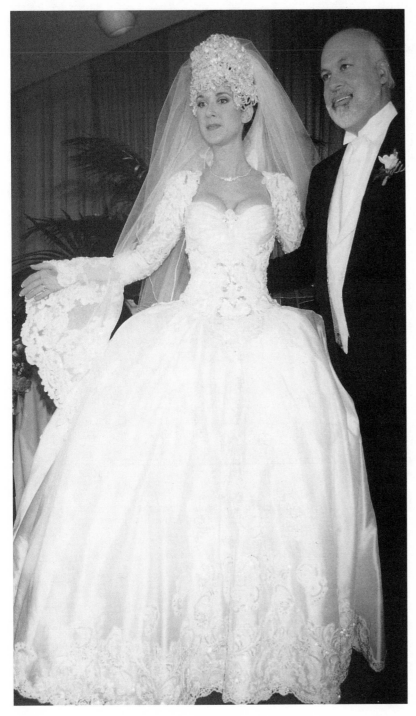

Inspired by eighteenth-century French court gowns, the satin and lace dress was embellished with hand-sewn pearls and a twenty-foot train. The combination of a low sweetheart neckline, flowing lace sleeves, and a basque waistline created an aura that was both feminine and regal.

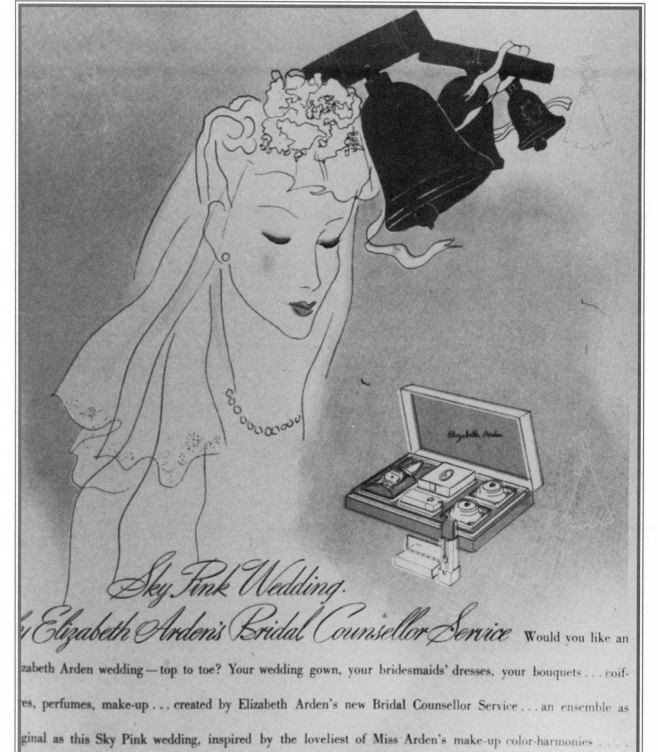

Sky Pink Wedding.

Elizabeth Arden's Bridal Counsellor Service Would you like an Elizabeth Arden wedding — top to toe? Your wedding gown, your bridesmaids' dresses, your bouquets . . . coiffures, perfumes, make-up . . . created by Elizabeth Arden's new Bridal Counsellor Service . . . an ensemble as original as this Sky Pink wedding, inspired by the loveliest of Miss Arden's make-up color-harmonies . . . .

PINK MAKE-UP HARMONY BOX, $5.50 • SKY PINK EVENING LIPSTICK, $2.00 • FLORAL BOUQUET OF 5 PERFUMES, $22.50 • SINGLE PERFUMES, $5.50

Elizabeth Arden

691 FIFTH AVENUE • NEW YORK

CHAPTER TWO

The Radiant Bridal Complexion and Smile

goals:
....

* **To identify skin strengths and weaknesses**
* **To establish a successful skin care plan**
* **To brighten a wedding day smile**

You deserve the sense of confidence that comes from knowing that your complexion is luminous and flawless. To get the skin you want, you need to develop a two-tier plan that cares for your individual skin type and corrects specific problems. To determine your skin type, pull back your hair and look at your skin, both in artificial and natural light. What do you see? Does it look dry? Oily? Are there reddish patches? Get out a piece of paper and start to write down your findings.

Identifying Your True Skin Profile

It's hard to overemphasize the importance of accurately determining your skin profile, but most women just react to what they see in the morning. If skin looks flaky, they use a moisturizer. If it looks oily, they scrub it with a strong soap. In fact, the skin you see in the mirror rarely shows the whole picture. It's been dried out with harsh soaps, drenched with moisturizers, burned by the sun, and chapped by cold winds. Read through all four skin profiles before you start making judgments. Answer every question carefully. Then count your answers. If you check off more than half of the questions in a particular profile, that's your skin profile.

Normal Skin

1. Your skin problems are minimal and mild; even as a teenager they were mild.
2. You need to wash your hair two to three times a week.
3. The surface of your skin is smooth and even, without reddened or flaky patches.
4. Your face has no enlarged pores or facial hair.
5. Your skin tans easily.

Dry Skin

1. Your skin has always been clear of acne.
2. Your hair seems to become drier between shampoos.
3. Your face feels taut after washing.
4. You are under thirty-five yet have fine lines around your eyes.
5. Powder tends to make your complexion look chalky.

Oily Skin

1. Your skin tends to break out.
2. You need to wash your hair every day.
3. Makeup wears off quickly.
4. Your skin tans evenly and easily.
5. Your mother looks years younger than her age.

Combination Skin

1. You have an oily nose and dry cheeks.
2. You have small bumps under your skin that never go away.
3. Sometimes there is dry, flaky, reddened skin around the nose.
4. Your hair may be drier in winter and oilier in summer.
5. You tend to burn, then tan in strong sunlight.

If you're not sure about your skin's strengths and weaknesses, try a three-day skin detoxification plan.

1. Declare a three-day moratorium on all the products that you routinely use on your hair and skin. This includes soaps, scrubbing grains, moisturizers, hand and body creams, regular shampoos and conditioners, and lip balm. You can still use mascara and lipstick.
2. Cleanse with liquid soapless soaps, such as Cytophil, or clear glycerine soaps, such as Neutrogena. Use this to wash your hands, face, and body.
3. Wash your hair with baby shampoo and do not use any conditioners.
4. Avoid sun exposure.

At the end of the three days, pull back your hair again and examine your skin in natural light.

* Does it look smooth and clear? You probably have normal skin.
* Does skin feel taut and tender? You probably have dry skin.
* Does your skin look oilier? The gentle soaps would not control your acne-prone skin; you probably have oily skin.
* Does your skin feel flaky around the nose, yet oily on chin and forehead? These are symptoms of combination skin.

If the skin profile questionnaire indicated a different type than you believed you had, be prepared for a remarkable change in the appearance of your skin as you follow a new skin care program.

Basic skin care follows three steps: a morning regimen to prepare the skin for makeup and protect it from pollution and sunlight; nighttime care to cleanse and correct the skin; and a weekly facial. For example, if your skin is oily, it is helpful to use scrubbing grains and alcohol-based toners. If your skin tends to be dry, nighttime care includes a moisturizer with vitamins and alpha-hydroxy acids. All skin types follow similar procedures, but which products are selected and how they are used varies according to individual skin profiles. Read the sections on different product formulations. Make notes that you can take with you to buy new beauty aids, jotting down key instructions and ingredients to look for.

Guide to Skin Care Products

The key to great skin care rests on selecting the right products for individual skin needs. There seems to be an endless variety of cleansers, toners, and moisturizers, but if you learn to recognize the basic different formulations, you will be able to make the best choices for any skin profile. You can learn a great deal about the products by reading both labels and instructions. For example, a moisturizer with a sunscreen would be designed for daytime use, since there is little exposure to strong light when you are asleep. Cleansers are best categorized by their instructions. If the label tells you that the formulation should be rinsed off with water, then it is a rinseable cleanser that does a wonderful job of removing soot and stale oil without leaving a greasy film. If it says the product should be massaged into the skin and then tissued off, it would be best for very dry complexions.

CLEANSERS

The role of a cleanser is to remove dry, old skin cells, stale oil, perspiration, and soot from the skin's surface. If skin is not thoroughly cleaned, it can look dull, flaky, reddened, and blotchy, and it will develop blackheads and blemishes. If the cleanser is too harsh, your skin will feel tight and look lined and rough.

Cold Cream:

Made of mineral oil, wax, and borax, cold cream is massaged into the skin, then tissued off. It removes dirt and loosens dry skin cells, but tends to leave an oily film on the face. It is a good start for dry skin, if you wear a heavy foundation, but will not provide adequate cleansing for other skin profiles.

Cleansing Creams:

Usually a combination of a cold cream base plus soaps or detergents, cleansing creams are rubbed into the skin and tissued off. They tend to leave a film of oil and soap on your skin that clogs pores and can make dry skin drier.

Rinseable Cream Cleansers:

Available in either cream or lotion formulations, rinseable cream cleansers are applied to the skin, massaged in lightly, then thoroughly rinsed off with water. They can work beautifully for all skin types, providing thorough but gentle cleansing.

Rinseable Gel Cleansers:

Wonderful cleansers for oily or acne-troubled skin, gel cleansers are designed to provide deep but nonirritating cleansing without using oils or wax that can provoke breakouts.

Abrasive Cleansers:

Available in tubes or pads, this gritty cleanser scrubs off dry skin and stale oil, leaving the skin smooth and fresh. They should not be used more than two to three times per week, to avoid excessive dryness and irritation.

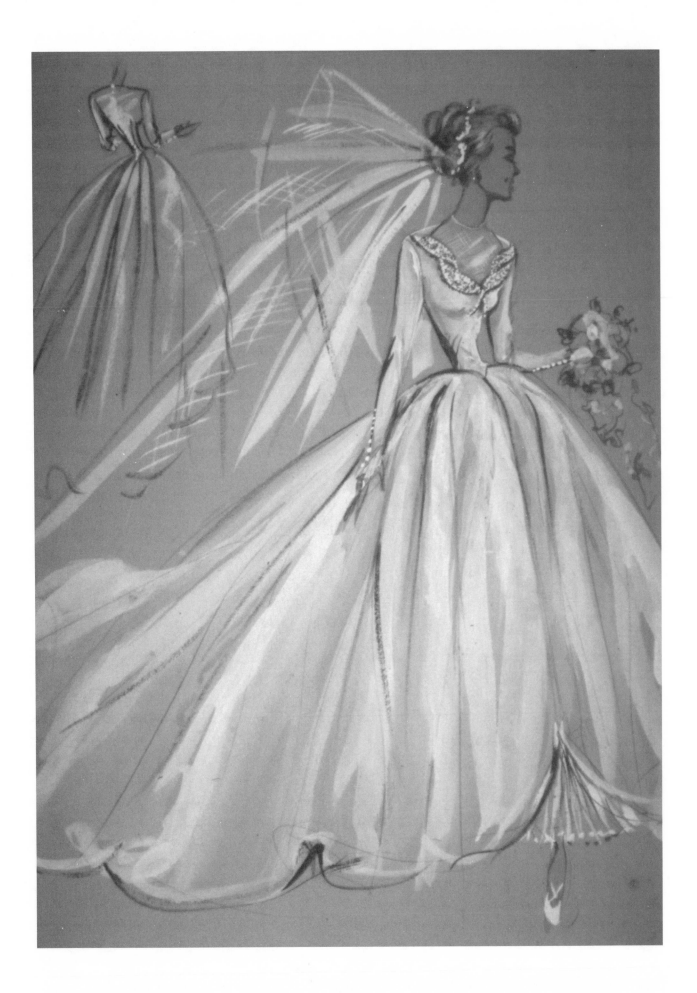

Recipes for Toners That You Can Make at Home

Homemade toners for all skin types are made of easily obtained ingredients. Mix all ingredients together in a bowl, transfer to a clean glass bottle, and store in the refrigerator.

NORMAL SKIN: Combine ¾ cup witch hazel, ¼ cup bottled water, and ½ teaspoon alum

OILY SKIN: Combine 1 cup witch hazel, ¼ teaspoon alum, 1 drop mint extract

COMBINATION/DRY SKIN: Combine 1 teaspoon each of dried chervil, rosemary, and thyme with ½ cup white wine. Bring to a boil, then steep for 30 minutes. Strain, then transfer to a clean glass bottle.

TONERS

Toning lotions are usually a mixture of water, alcohol, and glycerin, as well as a bit of color and fragrance. These traditional products refresh the skin after cleaning and prepare the surface for moisturizer and/or foundation. Depending on the formulation, they can diminish pores and remove traces of oil and dirt without causing unwanted dryness. They are good for all but drier skins. The impact on the skin can be varied by adding ingredients to stimulate circulation, soothe irritations, and diminish blemishes. They are used after cleansing and drying the face. There are three basic types:

Skin Fresheners:

Composed of alcohol, water, and detergent, they are excellent for normal to oily skin. A variety of additives such as allantoin or peppermint can provide different characteristics. Fresheners with allantoin soothe irritated skin while those with peppermint wake up circulation and produce a healthy glow to the skin.

Astringents:

Containing the same basic ingredients as fresheners, astringents tighten the skin, making fine lines and enlarged pores less visible. The most popular astringent uses witch hazel either singly or in combination with other ingredients. You can turn any skin freshener into an astringent by adding alum, found in the spice rack of a supermarket.

Clarifying Lotion:

This is the strongest type of toner, designed to make the skin look brighter and clearer by removing the top layer of dead skin cells. In addition to containing water, alcohol, and glycerin, clarifying lotions offer compounds like salicylic acids or fruit acids that break down dry hardened skin cells. They are effective for all but dry skin.

MOISTURIZERS

The traditional moisturizer uses a soothing mixture of oils, wax, and water to provide a protective film on the skin's surface to help it hold a healthy supply of water. High-tech moisturizers include an assortment of natural moisturizing factors such as hyaluronic acid, lactic acid, glycolic acid and glycosides that attract and hold water better and longer than traditional moisturizers. More benefits are achieved when sunscreens are added to reduce discoloration and skin aging.

Daytime Moisturizers:
Designed to be used under makeup, greaseless formulations are good for normal skin, while creamier products give drier skins the richness they need.

Night Creams or Moisturizers:
Heavier than daytime products, they should contain natural moisturizing factors in a richer base. They do not need a sunscreen. Such formulations are useful for dry skins, but may be too heavy for normal, oily, or combination skin types.

Anti-aging Moisturizers:
These sophisticated products are enriched with vitamins and/or hydroxy acids and sunscreens. The former reduce the appearance of fine lines, enlarged pores, and flaking skin, while the latter prevents sun-related aging.

Oil-free Moisturizers:
Compounded from water, emulsifiers, and natural moisturizing factors, they can smooth and brighten normal skin, which would not respond as well to heavier formulations.

Acne and Oil-Control "Reverse" Moisturizers:
Skin that becomes oily and is troubled by breakouts should use specially formulated gels and lotions to help clear pores and prevent blemishes. Usually containing benzoyl peroxide and/or salicylic acid, they remove the dulling film on the skin's surface that blocks the pores. The result? Skin looks fresh and soft without blemishes or an oily sheen.

FACE MASKS

The tightening and smoothing action of masks improves skin tone, texture, and color. They are to be used as part of a complete facial that includes cleansing and a facial sauna. Masks clarify the complexion, removing the top film on oily skin and helping dry skin regain a healthy water balance. There are two basic types.

Paste Masks:

These thick oatmeal- or clay-based formulations absorb excess oil, reduce inflammation, and rehydrate skin. Wonderful for oily, normal, or combination skin, they can be used in a weekly facial. Choose a commercial product or a homemade recipe provided in this chapter.

Gel Masks:

Clear and sticky, gel masks dry to a thin, smooth film. They rehydrate dry and normal skin, removing impurities and dry flaky skin. For greatest improvement they should be used regularly as part of a weekly facial. They are one of the easiest products to make yourself at home.

Skin Care 101

Each skin type should follow a daily morning and nighttime regimen and the bride should set aside time each week to do a complete facial. It will be time well spent. The procedure takes off the dulling film of stale oil and dead skin cells from the surface and feeds the skin essential moisture, leaving your skin smooth, bright, and clear. While a weekly facial is invaluable, you can still see a remarkable difference if facials are done every two to three weeks.

OILY SKIN

Oily skin needs thorough, nonirritating cleansing, mild drying agents, and oil-free formulations. It's important to avoid use of moisturizers, night creams, and creamy cleansers that can make oily skin look muddy and prone to breakouts. Clear glycerine soap, bar soaps with oatmeal, or liquid gel cleansers are all good cleansing choices. If the skin looks dull or feels sticky, you can use scrubbing cleansers that will remove the top layer of old, stale skin cells. After cleansing, a toner or astringent can freshen skin and shrink pores, as well as prepare the surface for oil-free foundation. If the oiliness is mild, use an alcohol-based freshener. If breakouts are a problem, use a freshener in the morning and a mild benzoyl peroxide lotion at night. Once a week, treat your skin to a deep-cleansing facial, complete with a mask.

Nighttime Care

1. If you use eye makeup, remove it with a nonoily eye makeup remover.
2. Wash face thoroughly with cleanser, massaging into skin to dissolve stale oil and loosen old, dead skin cells.
3. Rinse with four handfuls of warm water and two handfuls of cool—but not cold—water.
4. Dry face thoroughly.
5. Apply skin freshener or benzoyl peroxide.

Morning Care

1. Wash thoroughly with cleanser.
2. Dry face.
3. Dab on freshener with cotton ball.
4. Smooth on water-based foundation.

Weekly Facial

1. Remove eye makeup with nonoily cleanser.
2. Lather face with rinseable gel cleanser.
3. Steam face with parsley sauna.
4. Massage gently with abrasive cleanser.
5. Apply an oatmeal or clay mask for 10 minutes.
6. Rinse off with lukewarm, then cool, water.

Recipes for Face Masks That Can Be Made at Home

Face masks should be made fresh each time they are to be used. All ingredients should be combined in a small bowl and applied to the face with an unused ½-inch paint-brush. The masks should be allowed to harden and dry, usually fifteen to twenty minutes, then rinsed off with cool water.

NORMAL SKIN: Combine
1 egg white, 1 teaspoon honey,
1 teaspoon powdered milk,
1 pinch alum.

OILY SKIN: Combine 1 tablespoon rubbing alcohol, 2 tablespoons oatmeal, 1 teaspoon honey

COMBINATION SKIN: Mask A: Combine 1 egg yolk and 1 teaspoon honey; Mask B: combine 1 egg white and 1 tablespoon ground oatmeal. Spread Mask A on dry cheeks; use Mask B on forehead, nose, and chin.

DRY SKIN: Combine
1 tablespoon full-fat yogurt,
1 egg yolk, 1 teaspoon honey,
1 teaspoon mayonnaise.

NORMAL SKIN

The basic rule for normal skin is: First, do no harm. Do not use harsh soaps that will dry it out, or drown it in oily moisturizers that could promote breakouts. It responds beautifully to creamy, rinseable cleansers, nondrying

The Skin-Smoothing Sauna

The warm, fragrant steam of a facial sauna stimulates circulation, lifts away dead dry skin, and offers a source of moisture to thirsty skin.

The equipment couldn't be simpler: a one-gallon cooking pot, a large towel, and a lemon or selection of dried herbs. For each sauna, fill a pot with water and bring it to a boil. Add herbs or lemon slices and simmer for five minutes. Remove from heat and place it on a solid table. Sit in front of the pot and drape a towel over your head to capture steam. Stay under the towel for three to five minutes. If it feels too warm, lift up the towel and take in a few gulps of fresh air, then duck back under the towel to finish the sauna. It is one of the safest and easiest home-based beauty techniques, as long as the pot of the hot water is placed on a steady table.

Saunas should be part of a complete facial. They should be done regularly up to the last week before the wedding. As the date approaches, skin care should be especially gentle to avoid any unanticipated problems.

toners, and oil-free moisturizers fortified with alpha-hydroxy exfoliators, and sunscreens for protection. In addition to a morning and nighttime routine, a weekly cleansing and hydrating facial keeps normal skin balanced and beautiful.

Nighttime Care

1. Remove eye makeup with nonoily remover pads.
2. Use warm—but not hot—water, to avoid damaging blood vessels.
3. Twice a week, use scrubbing grains or pads, instead of regular cleanser.
4. If skin feels tight, use an oil-free alpha-hydroxy moisturizer on cheeks, but avoid nose, chin, and forehead.

Morning Care

1. Wash face with rinseable cleanser.
2. Freshen skin with toner applied with cotton ball.
3. Allow face to dry.
4. Apply oil-free sunscreen or foundation fortified with sunblock.

Weekly Facial

1. Remove eye makeup.
2. Wash face with rinseable cleanser.
3. Steam face with rosemary facial sauna.
4. Massage very gently with mild abrasive cleansing pads that have been moistened with water.
5. Smooth a mask over the face staying well away from the eye area. If your skin feels a little tight, choose a gel or moisturizing mask. If your skin feels irritated or oily, use a clear oatmeal mask. Apply a commercial mask, or use one of the recipes provided in this chapter.

The Eighteenth-Century Bride

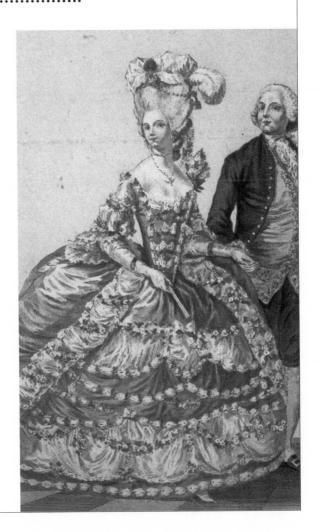

A bride at the time of Louis XVI reddened her cheeks with a rough pad saturated with rouge called Spanish Red. Rouge was so popular at the court that a French finance minister suggested taxing rouge pots to raise revenue to provide funds for soldiers' widows.

Beauty standards called for a doll-like appearance with whitened skin, bright circles of rouge on the cheeks, and darkened eyebrows. If white powder did not provide the desired porcelain surface, women might attach leeches to their cheeks to reduce natural blush.

Their hair was an engineering marvel. Supported by wires and padding and coated with pomade and powder, a typical wedding style was a combination of curls, tendrils, loops, and waves.

DRY SKIN

There are probably more products and treatments designed for dry skin than for any other beauty problem. In reality, dry skin simply needs only five basic products: a mild, creamy, rinseable cleanser that removes dirt without dehydrating the skin, an alcohol-free toner to freshen the skin, an alpha-hydroxy–enriched night cream to promote cell renewal, a vitamin- and sunscreen-fortified daytime moisturizer that protects against aging UV rays, and a hydrating mask to smooth out lines and skin tone. A weekly facial enhances the good care provided by daily cleansing and moisturizing. Avoid bar soaps, which can leave the skin red and irritated, cold cream cleansers, which leave an oily film on the face, and alcohol-based toners, which dehydrate the skin.

Nighttime Care

1. Remove eye makeup with nonoily remover.
2. Wet face and hands and massage a nickel-sized dollop of creamy, rinseable cleanser into cheeks, forehead, chin, and nose.
3. Rinse off thoroughly with ten handfuls of warm water. Pat face with towel.
4. If you are using a vitamin-based moisturizer, apply it immediately to your slightly damp face. If you are using a hydroxy moisturizer, wait a few minutes before applying it to avoid irritation.

Morning Care

1. Repeat nighttime cleansing.
2. Dab on moisturizing astringent with fresh cotton ball.
3. Allow face to dry before applying a sunscreen enriched moisturizer.
4. Allow it to absorb before applying an oil-rich foundation.

Weekly Facial

1. Remove eye makeup with nonoily eye makeup remover.
2. Cleanse with rich, rinseable formulation.
3. Steam face with lavender facial for five minutes.
4. Rinse off with cold water.
5. Apply rich moisturizing mask for ten minutes.
6. Rinse off mask.
7. Apply moisturizer to skin.

COMBINATION SKIN

Combination skin is never boring. At the beginning of the week, your skin can feel tight and dry. By Wednesday, you may wake with a few unappreciated blemishes. To stay ahead of your skin's shape-shifting tendencies, start skin care with a rinseable gel liquid cleanser, to do a thorough but nondrying job. Dab a low-alcohol freshener on forehead, nose, and chin, and a high-tech, oil-free moisturizer on the cheeks. Choose a product that uses alpha- or beta-hydroxy compounds to hydrate the skin, rather than a heavy, oily formulation. Have a mild benzoyl peroxide gel on hand to dab on periodic breakouts. Don't use abrasive cleansers, which may provoke problems in oily areas and dehydrate drier ones.

Nighttime Care

1. Remove eye makeup with nonoily eye makeup remover.
2. Cleanse face with rinseable gel cleanser formulated for normal skin.
3. Rinse with five handfuls of warm and four handfuls of cool water.
4. Dab toner on chin, nose, and forehead.
5. With cotton ball, apply high-tech moisturizer only on dry areas.
6. If there are breakouts, dab them with a mild benzoyl peroxide gel.

Morning Care

1. Wash face with gel rinseable cleanser.
2. Freshen skin with alcohol toner.
3. Apply oil-free sunscreen or light foundation that contains sunscreen.

Weekly Facial

1. Remove eye makeup with nonoily makeup remover.
2. Steam for four minutes with lemon sauna.
3. Gently massage center of face with a dampened abrasive sponge.
4. Rinse off with five handfuls of warm water and five handfuls of cool—but not cold—water.
5. Apply oatmeal mask in center of face, and gel mask on cheeks. Leave on for ten minutes.
6. Rinse off with warm water, and pat your face dry.

The Ten Major Skin Problems and How to Eliminate Them

In addition to the problems inherent with each skin type there are problems that can occur in a range of skin types. Fortunately, there are simple and quick solutions that can be easily done prior to a wedding.

PROBLEM #1:
BREAKOUTS AND BLEMISHES

Nobody needs to take a test to judge if they have acne-prone skin. We all know the lumps, bumps, and blackheads that appear without warning to sabotage a perfect hair day or a fabulous dress. Because blemishes are a direct result of unwanted oil production, traditional treatments call for an endless round of drying soaps, toners, and masks. The result: Dry, flaky skin and breakouts.

New developments and products have led to a far more effective choice of remedies. If eruptions are small and infrequent, use a rinseable gel cleanser, astringent, and benzoyl peroxide gel both morning and night. Keep blemishes under control with an oil-free foundation and avoid all moisturizers. Start using benzoyl peroxide twice a day, until eruptions subside; then use it only at night. Try this program for two weeks. If blemishes persist, your skin needs help only available from a dermatologist. They can start by prescribing oral antibiotics to eliminate pore-attacking bacteria.

If your skin still is troubled by acne, doctors may prescribe a gel form of vitamin A known as Retin-A. Just a few drops, spread over the face, peels off skin cells that cover the pores and literally empties the follicles of acne-provoking oil. Retin-A is not without side effects. It can be very irritating and many women notice their skin looks very flushed. In the first few weeks of treatment, your skin may look a little worse, because the Retin-A is bringing to the surface eruptions that were going to occur over the next few months. When using Retin-A, it is important to stay out of the sun, since the powerful acne fighters cause increased sun sensitivity. Retin-A is usually used twice a day to eliminate and prevent acne problems. If this proves to be too irritating, you can use benzoyl peroxide gel in the morning, and Retin-A only at night. The rest of your skin care routine needs to be extremely gentle. Use a mild, rinseable oil-free cleanser, and avoid any type of toner, astringent, or scrubbing grains. Dry lips can be soothed with medicated lip balm.

Severe, persistent acne with large blemishes and hard cysts responds well to an oral form of Retin-A called Accutane. It is a powerful weapon that can actually cure severe, persistent acne problems in about six months. Doctors believe it works by permanently shutting down oil glands. In other words, no oil, no acne. Accutane is not for everyone. Some women develop very dry, cracked lips, body aches, and peeling of the palms of the hands and the soles of the feet. More significant, Accutane has been linked to serious birth defects. Before starting the drug, it is essential to take a pregnancy test to avoid harming a baby. To be safe, most doctors like their patients to wait six months after ending Accutane therapy before planning pregnancy. Finally, Accutane increases sun sensitivity, so plan on ending treatment at least a month before a sun-drenched honeymoon to avoid problems. When using Accutane, cleanse your face with a very mild, rinseable cleanser. Avoid astringents, abrasive cleansers, and masks. Sunscreens and lip balm should be part of the daily skin care routine.

PROBLEM #2: FRECKLES

Adorable on a snub-nosed six-year-old, a bride may feel that freckles aren't nearly as charming with a formal white wedding gown. To manage freckles, you need to use a two-step process. A lightening technique erases existing freckles, and a commitment to sunscreens prevents new freckles from forming. Look for lightening creams and gels that contain both hydroquinone and a sunscreen, which blocks melanin production; as dark-tone cells age and fall off the skin, new skin cells are fresh and clear. The sunscreen prevents new freckles from developing. These products take time—usually three months to show significant change in the skin. A more dramatic change can be achieved with a Yag laser, which literally vaporizes the top layer of freckled skin cells. The skin is anesthetized and the laser light pulses burn off the freckled skin. The next day the skin becomes crusted and reddened; the redness will last up to six weeks. Sunscreen must be used all the time to protect the skin and prevent new freckles.

Laser-Based Skin Care

At the frontier of modern skin care, laser skin resurfacing literally erases the skin's imperfections. Lasers emit a powerful and focused light that smooths scars, fine lines, freckles, and even destroys unwanted facial hair.

According to New York dermatologist Albert Lefkovits there are several types of lasers, each with its own set of strengths and weaknesses. "The CO2 laser is used for resurfacing deeply lined and wrinkled skin, while the ruby or YAG laser works beautifully for freckles and hair removal," he explained. The skin is first numbed and the laser beam is directed to the trouble spots. After treatment, the skin becomes reddened and is covered with thick ointments to promote healing. After seven to ten days, the skin looks smooth, albeit slightly reddened. Because healing time can be so long, it is wise to schedule the last laser treatment three months before the wedding.

For best results, it is vital that laser therapy be performed by a dermatologist or cosmetic surgeon trained in the technique, because scarring and discoloration have resulted from unskilled operators. "Latino, Asian, and African-American complexion tones are at a higher risk of incurring dark or light patches from laser resurfacing," notes Dr. Lefkovits, chairman of a recent symposium on laser therapy held at Mt. Sinai Medical School. "To avoid problems, always test a laser on your arm or leg before aiming it at your face. If the redness goes away within twenty-four hours, you are a good candidate for this high-tech skin care. If the skin stays red for days and/or the area looks lighter or darker than the surrounding skin, lasers are probably not for you."

PROBLEM #3: BROKEN BLOOD VESSELS

The thin, fine red lines that appear around the nose and cheeks are actually small ruptured blood vessels. Overaggressive facial massage, too hot saunas, and heavy drinking can rupture small vessels, particularly in thin, sensitive skin. Whatever the cause, this is one of the simplest problems to erase. A dermatologist painlessly zaps a ruptured vessel with a cauterizing needle. This seals off additional bleeding, and the line vanishes. The treatment leaves a tiny scab, which falls off in a day. There may be residual redness for a week, so it should not be done less than a month before the wedding.

PROBLEM #4: BROWN PATCHES

Irregular, darkened patches make the skin look dull and muddy. They can appear during pregnancy, in reaction to birth control pills, and as an after-effect of a bad sunburn. Frequently, several months of Retin-A or glycolic acid peels will remove discolored skin and reveal fresh, clear texture. Because Retin-A tends to make the skin look flushed, plan a three-month treatment at least four months before the wedding. Alternatively, skin tones can be evened out with a resurfacing laser. For safety and good results, the lasers should be tested on an inconspicuous spot such as the inside of a thigh. If the skin heals easily and there are no unwanted changes in skin color, you can proceed with confidence. Like all laser treatments, topical anesthetic is used just prior to treatment and redness can persist for up to six weeks.

PROBLEM #5: CROW'S-FEET

Fine lines around the eyes are a sign of life that is well lived. They come from laughing with friends, and long lazy days in the sun. Many women find that three to four months' of applying Retin-A to the area smooths out the lines. It is felt that Retin-A helps the body to restore collagen, which fills up the lines around the eyes. When the lines are deep and numerous, dermatologists can inject Botox to relax the muscles that are wrinkling the skin. The effects last four to six months. Botox can also be used to relax frown lines on the forehead and between the eyes. Botox is actually derived from the toxin produced from the botulinus bacteria, which can cause a type of fatal food poisoning, but, as horrible as it sounds, it's injected locally in the skin and is not absorbed by the rest of the body.

PROBLEM #6: SCARS

The aftereffects of acne include enlarged pores, discolorations, and skin depressions, as well as raised, lumpy scar tissue. If these problems are fairly mild, dermatologists may try a series of six to eight glycolic peels to refine the skin's surface. These glycolic peels are much stronger than the products available in the stores. They are a 70 percent solution, whereas the strongest solution that you can buy in a drug- or department store is about 12 percent. When the problems are more significant, the entire surface can be treated with dermabrasion, a motor-driven wire brush that rubs off the top layer of affected skin. For this procedure, the skin is anesthetized. Crusting and healing takes about eight to ten days, while redness can persist for four to six weeks. More recently, dermatologists have been using laser treatments to resurface and remove acne and other scars.

PROBLEM #7: SENSITIVE SKIN

Does your skin tend to become reddened, itchy, or break out in a rash? Does it burn easily or rarely tan? It probably doesn't come as much of a surprise for you to learn that you have sensitive skin. To keep sensitive skin under control, you need nonirritating products and treatments to prevent problems, as well as an assortment of remedies to relieve your skin if it becomes irritated. Studies have shown that half of all allergic reactions are due to the perfumes products contain, so fragrance-free products are a good choice for easily annoyed skin. Also avoid abrasive cleansing, toners with alcohol, and both alpha- and beta-hydroxy acids. Sensitive skin does well with oatmeal soaps and masks. When skin does become inflamed, Benadryl or calamine lotion or over-the-counter steroids will relieve redness and inflammation. Nobody wants to wake up with itchy, blotchy skin. But for a bride, it can cast a pall over a carefully planned wedding day. If you have reactive skin, be very selective of the products you use around the time of your wedding. Never use a new, untried beauty aid; select only those that have worked well in the past. If your face and chest tend to become red and splotchy with stress, consider a wedding gown with a high neckline.

PROBLEM #8:
DARK UNDER-EYE CIRCLES

The thin, under-eye skin tends to reflect the bluish tones in the underlying blood vessels. You may notice that when you're tired or ill, the shadows under your eyes become darker and deeper. Actually, under stress, the face looks paler and the contrast is greater between the face and the under-eye areas. A soothing mask that increases circulation can reduce pallor and make under-eye shadows less apparent. In some women, dark circles are an inherited tendency, thought to be due to an increased production of melanin. Wearing a sunscreen and oversized sunglasses will prevent exposure and dramatically decrease under-eye dark circles.

PROBLEM #9: SWOLLEN EYES

Puffy eye skin above and below the eyes are often due to chronic allergies. If your eyes seem swollen when you wake up, try taking a decongestant before going to sleep. Raising the head of the bed a few inches will also help drain the excess fluid from blood vessels around the eyes. Put a brick under each side of the head of the bed to discourage fluid buildup. Puffiness can be relieved with cold tea bags, offering both tannin and coolness, which tighten swollen tissues.

If allergies have been a long-term problem, the skin around the eyes becomes permanently puffy and stretched out, creating an aging and tired expression. In this situation, eye packs will not provide relief. A cosmetic surgery procedure called blepharoplasty will remove excess skin from the upper and lower lids. This surgery is usually done as part of an overall face lift, but when the eyes are prematurely aged, blepharoplasty can be done alone with good results.

PROBLEM #10: ENLARGED PORES

The much maligned pore is the usually invisible hole through which oil released by the glands reaches the skin's surface. If the oil glands have been very busy, the excess oil production tends to stretch the pore opening to the point of visibility. If you control oiliness, the enlarged pores should not become a problem. If they are already a problem, both alpha-hydroxy acids and Retin-A can empty clogged, distended pores of excess oil and debris. After several weeks of treatment, these powerful skin care tools will refine your skin's surface and diminish pore size.

Follow the skin care program for oily skin, but eliminate use of astringents and scrubbing grains. Apply Retin-A cream or an alpha-hydroxy gel formulated for acne in a thin layer over the entire face. Avoid using any moisturizers—and even oil-free sunscreens—until skin texture improves. If you use Retin-A, be sure to avoid sun exposure.

Bridal Skin Care Product List

★ Soap or rinseable cleanser
★ Scrubbing grains
★ Toner
★ Daytime moisturizer with sunscreen
★ Nighttime moisturizer with lactic or glycolic acid
  (for all but oily and acne-prone skins)
★ Antioil and blemish gel for problem skin
★ Face masks
★ Clean washcloths
★ Cotton balls
★ Large pot and bath towel
★ Dried herbs and fresh lemons for facial sauna

As you work to develop your most successful skin care routines, make note of the products that do the best job. Set up a box to hold your wedding day beauty supplies. As you identify the cleansers, toners, moisturizers, and the like that give you the results you want, buy a fresh bottle, label it, and place it in the box. Don't even think of using it before the day of the ceremony.

The Dazzling Bridal Smile

On the wedding day, a bride wants a smile that expresses all the happiness that she feels. If her teeth are discolored, chipped, or oddly shaped or spaced, even the most confident bride may feel self-conscious. Happily, new dental techniques and products are now available that quickly and safely produce a more beautiful and radiant smile.

The first step to a more beautiful smile is a thorough cleaning and polishing. A dental hygienist will remove dulling plaque from the tooth's surface and edges below the gum line, and polish the surface with a gently abrasive paste or salt water spray. In less than forty-five minutes, the clean teeth will feel fresh, smooth and look brighter.

After a cleaning, a dentist can examine the mouth to make a list of minor adjustments that will create a major improvement. According to New York–based dentist Myron Finkel, a beautiful smile is a symmetrical smile. "When I look at a bride-to-be, I look first at the size and shape of the teeth. With a sanding disc I can shorten long teeth, even off chips, smooth off ragged edges, and round off edges for a more feminine smile," he explained.

If the cleaning and polishing did not remove all the discoloration, the surface can be bleached with a peroxide compound to a bright, dazzling white with a choice of three techniques. If the wedding is less than six weeks away, the entire mouth can be lightened in a single session. A peroxide solution is applied to the front upper and lower teeth and an energizing light is aimed at the mouth to hasten chemical reaction. At the end of a forty-five-minute session, the teeth are rinsed off. This technique works well, but may be too intense for teeth that are sensitive or damaged.

Many dentists, including Dr. Finkel, prefer a dentist-assisted home care bleaching program. "At the first visit, we make a mold for the upper and/or lower teeth," he explained. "At the second visit, we give the patient a two-week supply of bleaching product that is to be used at night. The lightening compound is placed in the custom-made tray and slipped into the mouth. After two weeks of nightly use, the difference is remarkable. You will need four weeks—two weeks for each side—to bleach both top and bottom."

Commercially available home kits use the same materials in a mouth tray. They are far less expensive but are not as effective. Part of the problem is the tray, which is sold in a one-size-fits-all kit. If it doesn't fit properly, it may not create enough contact with the bleaching product to produce the desired lightening effect.

When bleaching and shaping still leave problems, laminates can cover each tooth with a translucent glass nail. Custom-fitted and tinted, it can hide dark stains, fill in chips, and close up spaces between the teeth. Laminates can be used to cover a single tooth, or applied to several or even all of the front teeth. Taking at least two visits to complete each tooth, it is a long-lasting (about ten years with good care), albeit time-consuming and expensive procedure.

Bonding is a less expensive and somewhat quicker cosmetic dental technique that applies a plastic tooth-colored material to the surface of the tooth. The dentist can work on two to three teeth per visit, using bonding to cover discolorations, fill in chips, and close up gaps between teeth. It takes about forty-five minutes per visit, lasts up to three years, and is one tenth as expensive as laminates. Once your teeth are bonded, it is best to avoid foods that stain, including cherries, coffee, and beets. Care should be taken when biting into corn on the cob and bagels, to avoid breakage.

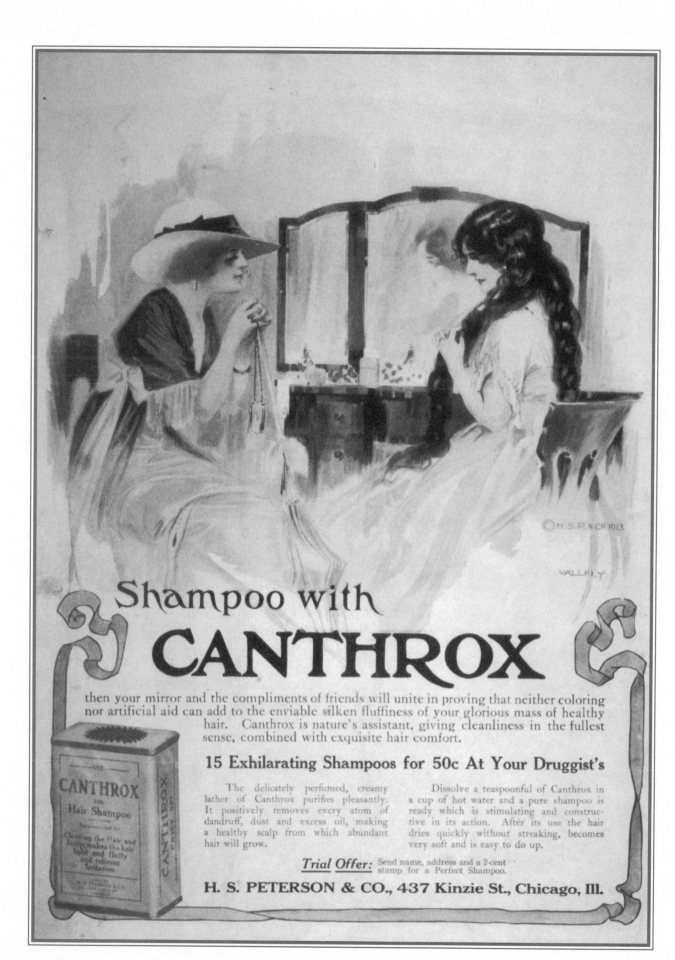

Shampoo with
CANTHROX

then your mirror and the compliments of friends will unite in proving that neither coloring nor artificial aid can add to the enviable silken fluffiness of your glorious mass of healthy hair. Canthrox is nature's assistant, giving cleanliness in the fullest sense, combined with exquisite hair comfort.

15 Exhilarating Shampoos for 50c At Your Druggist's

The delicately perfumed, creamy lather of Canthrox purifies pleasantly. It positively removes every atom of dandruff, dust and excess oil, making a healthy scalp from which abundant hair will grow.

Dissolve a teaspoonful of Canthrox in a cup of hot water and a pure shampoo is ready which is stimulating and constructive in its action. After its use the hair dries quickly without streaking, becomes very soft and is easy to do up.

Trial Offer: Send name, address and a 2-cent stamp for a Perfect Shampoo.

H. S. PETERSON & CO., 437 Kinzie St., Chicago, Ill.

CHAPTER THREE

The Bride's Crowning Glory

goals:
....
★ **To understand the different hair characteristics**

★ **To develop a successful hair care program**

Wedding hair styles begin with healthy shining, soft hair that glows with rich, bright color.

Beautiful Healthy Hair

The earlier you start caring properly for your hair, the better; even two months of intensive conditioning can make a remarkable difference.

CHOOSING THE RIGHT SHAMPOO

For beautiful hair, whether it is dry, normal, or oily, start with the appropriate shampoo. You want a formulation that will thoroughly remove dirt and stale oil, yet preserve moisture and texture. While all shampoos are composed primarily of detergents, oils, wax, and water, they can be modified depending on the qualities and quantities of additional ingredients.

Protein Shampoos:
Proteins adhere to hair strands, adding strength and restoring flexibility. Protein fills in cracks in the cuticle caused by coloring, waving, and straightening. Because it completely coats the hair strand, a protein shampoo makes the hair look thicker and fuller. All hair types and textures (except bushy or curly hair) respond beautifully to protein-rich shampoos.

Sunscreen Shampoos:

The same PABA and cinnamates that are used in skin care products can be added to shampoos and conditioners. They can prevent some of the disintegration associated with the actual rays of the sun, but cannot prevent dehydration from the sun's heat. Sunscreen-fortified shampoos can be helpful if you live in a sunny climate, but should not give you a false sense of security. If you are going to spend more than fifteen minutes in direct sun, cover your head with scarf or hat.

Baby Shampoos:

Originally created to avoid eye irritation, they are designed to cleanse sparse, fine baby hair. They can work well as a daily shampoo if your hair is short, thin, or somewhat dry, but may not provide adequate cleansing for longer, thicker, or oilier hair.

Vitamin Shampoos:

Although a whole alphabet of vitamins have been added to shampoos, to date only a form of vitamin B6, called panthenol, has proven to be absorbable by the hair shaft. Panthenol permeates the hair shaft and appears to restructure damaged or brittle hair.

Everyday Shampoos:

Formulated to be used every day, these shampoos are usually mild detergents enriched with small amounts of conditioning agents. If you have oily hair or use styling gels or mousse, it may not offer enough cleansing, even if used everyday.

Silk Shampoos:

Almost microscopic strips of silk fibers in a shampoo can add a wonderful shine and finish. Silk does not heal damaged hair, but acts like hundreds of tiny mirrors to reflect light. It can add a glorious brightness to normal, curly, and bushy hair.

Chemically Damaged Hair Shampoos:

Hair that has been colored, permed, or straightened has been subjected to alkaline formulations necessary to change the color or texture of the hair. The processing products roughen and weaken hair strands, creating a need for shampoos to restore strength and softness. A properly formulated shampoo for chemically damaged hair should offer a low pH to shrink swollen hair strands, protein to provide a protective coating, and humectant to restore moisture.

pH-balanced Shampoos:

Soaps and shampoos have a naturally alkaline pH. For healthy or oily hair, this will not cause a problem. When hair is dry, coarse, or chemically treated, an alkaline pH can leave the hair thin, brittle, and lifeless. To keep hair soft and lively, look for a balanced- or low-pH shampoo to add strength and shine.

CONDITIONERS

The best time to use a conditioner is before you need it to prevent damage, rather than once the hair starts to look dry and feel stiff. Most women should regularly use two to three different types of conditioners, depending on their hair type and texture. Conditioners restore flexibility as they prevent breakage and split ends.

Creme Rinse:

One of the first commercial conditioners, these pearly lotions use alum salts to temporarily relax and soften the hair strand. They are wonderful for coarse, bushy hair texture, but are not helpful for thin, brittle, or damaged hair. Stir a tablespoon into a cup of warm water after a shampoo, then rinse out thoroughly. If the hair has a tendency to be wiry, combine two tablespoons of creme rinse to two tablespoons of hot water.

Instant Conditioners:

Composed primarily of waxes and proteins, these products are applied to freshly washed hair and left on for no more than two minutes, then rinsed off. These products coat the hair shaft with a protein/polymer film that adds shine and flexibility. They can also help prevent problems in hair that is styled with a hair dryer. They are a quick and effective choice for all but the oiliest hair textures.

Every Bride Is Beautiful

Deep Conditioners:

Rich in proteins and oils, these thick, creamy conditioners remain on the head for thirty to forty minutes, usually under a heat cap. They are designed for hair showing signs of damage from coloring, waving, straightening, or blow-drying. They provide protein and moisture to restore strength, flexibility, and shine. They should be used on a regular schedule, a week after chemically treating your hair. They are helpful to all hair types and textures that are subjected to processing.

Hot Oil Conditioners:

Clear formulations of oil and water, these are heated slightly then worked through the hair. They are wonderful for naturally dry hair, which seems to get drier between shampoos. Dryness due to processing is best handled by deep conditioners.

Leave-in Conditioners:

Depending on the formulation, these products add body, restore shine, or smooth split ends. They are particularly helpful for frizzy or heat-damaged hair.

Choosing and using the right shampoo and conditioner depends on the individual needs of your hair. To banish bad hair days, it is important to identify hair strengths and weaknesses, selecting a range of products and techniques for the results you want.

The Basics of Beautiful Hair

When you are planning a skin care program, you need to simply identify the type. With hair care, you need to identify the three *T*s: type, texture, and tone.

There are three basic hair types: oily, normal, and dry. Oily hair tends to stick together and look limp by the end of the day. It tends to lose style quickly, with curls and body fading within a few hours. Things seem to get worse in the summer, and dandruff is a frequent problem. Oily hair needs daily low-oil shampoos and a lemon juice rinse. It's important to avoid creamy conditioners, creme rinses, and oily gels.

Naturally dry hair looks dull and feels stiff. It seems to become drier and bushier between shampoos, and resists attempts to curl and style. It is often accompanied by dry scalp dandruff. Dry hair needs gentle but thorough shampoos and a creme rinse to add softness and shine.

Normal hair is healthy and balanced with a natural shine, stays fresh between shampoos, and takes curl and style easily. Dandruff flakes are rare. Normal hair is usually "virgin hair," unprocessed hair that has never been treated with coloring, waving, or straightening solutions. Good care for normal hair includes shampoos and conditioners formulated for healthy, strong hair. The cleansing should be thorough, but nondrying. The right shampoo leaves the hair shiny, soft, and manageable. Conditioners can be a simple creme rinse or an instant protein formulation. Deep conditioners that remain on the head for fifteen to twenty minutes are too heavy and will leave the hair limp.

THE TRUTH ABOUT HAIR TEXTURE

It is hard to overestimate the importance of hair texture to overall appearance of the hair.

Fine texture tends to look flat and sparse and is usually a problem of oily hair. There are average numbers of hair, but each strand is noticeably thin. It is good to use a shampoo without conditioners designed for oily hair, and avoid all conditioners, rinses, and heavy hair sprays, which will flatten fine hair. While the hair is still damp from the shampoo, you can build in volume by distributing a mousse throughout the hair before styling.

Coarse hair is hair with attitude. Thick and wiry, this is strong hair with its own agenda. Its coarse texture tends to be full, bushy, and hard to style. This hair needs a shampoo rich in conditioners, a good creme rinse to relax the hair strands, and weekly deep conditioning to maintain moisture and flexibility. A light dab of finishing oil after styling will restore shine and provide control. Avoid hairstyles with bangs, since they will curl up and defy you. If you want to straighten your hair, don't use a chemical relaxer more than twice a year—and never in conjunction with hair coloring. Wait at least two weeks between procedures.

Naturally curly texture is thick and healthy with body to spare, but at the slightest sign of humidity, the pretty curls turn into a bushy frizz. Care includes rich conditioning shampoos, creme rinses, and a silicone finishing lotion to protect the strands from frizz-provoking moisture. To soften the hair without weighing it down, try an electric brush to temporarily relax the strands. It works quickly with less damage than would occur straightening curly hair with a hair dryer and paddle brush.

RECOGNIZING HAIR TONE

Hair tone refers to the strength, flexibility, and shine of the hair. If your hair looks dull and stiff, yet you don't color or wave your hair, your hair strands may be covered by a layer of dirt and oil that is not adequately removed when you shampoo. Try a shampoo product for oily hair and rinse for a full minute under the shower to flush out every trace of cleanser. Finish off the shampoo with a lemon juice rinse. If the hair seems dry, use a light creme rinse, primarily toward the ends of the hair, and rinse out thoroughly. If the color remains dull, try highlights around the face to brighten overall impact.

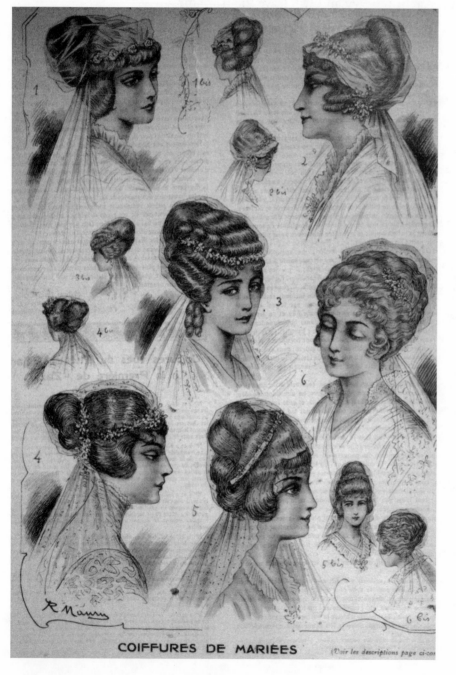

COIFFURES DE MARIÉES

(Voir les descriptions page ci-co...

Stiff, flyaway hair tone is a not uncommon side effect of coloring, waving, or straightening the hair. The chemicals used to get the job done alter the physical properties in the hair strand. It seems almost unfair that a beautiful, new color or texture is accompanied by a stiff, dry appearance. To avoid trading one problem for another, condition before shampoos, use shampoos designed to strengthen processed hair, avoid swimming in salt water or chlorinated pools, and protect your hair from exposure to the sun with a hat. Every ten days, let your hair dry naturally, without a hair dryer or rollers. Once a week, set aside thirty minutes for a deep, intensive conditioning, and trim your hair frequently to avoid split ends.

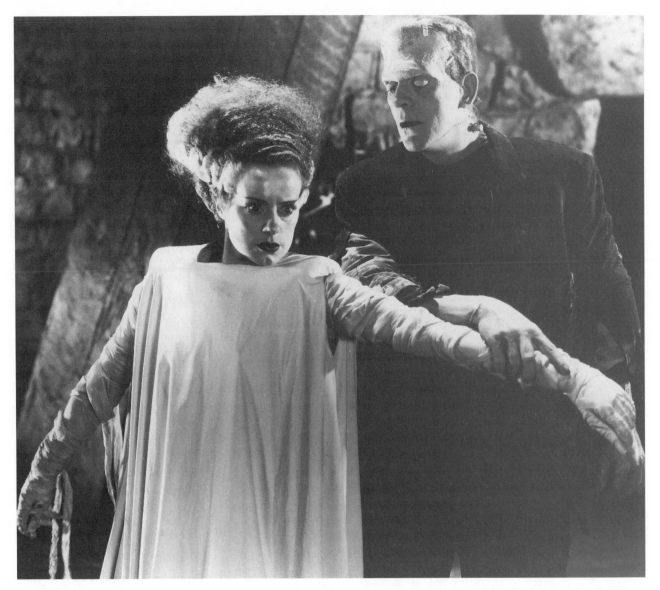

The Hair You Don't Want

Intensive Conditioning Treatment

1. Whip together ½ cup low-fat mayonnaise, 1 egg yolk, 1 tablespoon soft margarine, and 2 teaspoons wheat germ oil.
2. Apply to hair and scalp, completely covering each strand with a thick layer of conditioner.
3. Soak a terry-lined shower cap in hot water, wring out, and pull over head.
4. Allow this conditioning cap to remain on the head for thirty to forty-five minutes.
5. Remove the cap. You'll be surprised how much conditioner your thirsty, dry hair has absorbed.
6. Wash out the residual conditioner and allow hair to air dry or use a dryer set on cool.

Every Bride Is Beautiful

43

Brittle tone has a damaged, strawlike appearance. It tends to look dull and rough and seems to be getting thinner. This hair needs a rest. Avoid straightening or permanent waving. If possible, stop coloring your hair. Use a shampoo for processed hair, a protein-rich conditioner, and avoid or eliminate hair dyes, hot rollers, curling irons, or hot combs. Use an intensive deep conditioning each week to restore strength, shine, and flexibility. Choose a commercial product or use the recipes in this chapter.

If your hair doesn't respond to four weeks of intensive conditioning and gentle care, cutting off the damaged hair may be the best option. It is a hard choice for a bride to make, but it is a decision best made early enough for healthy regrowth. The alternative is an unwanted short haircut just before the wedding.

The Three Leading Hair and Scalp Problems

In many ways hair is much more predictable than your skin. In addition to problems that are unique to individual hair characteristics, there are universal issues that pop up often when they are least welcome.

PROBLEM #1: DANDRUFF

Blond or brunette, short or long, dry or oily, every hair type and texture can develop annoying flakes of dandruff. We are always shedding scalp cells as old cells die and new ones are formed. When the scalp is healthy and well balanced, the changeover is imperceptible. When the scalp becomes too dry or oily, or if the rate of growth is disrupted, the cells clump together and fall off in visible flakes. For oily hair conditions, a sulfur-based dandruff shampoo will both slow down oil gland production on the scalp and break up dandruff cells. They are best used just until dandruff is under control, and then once a week, rather than as regular shampoo. When the scalp is dry, dandruff flakes are piling up because of dehydration. Use a dry scalp dandruff shampoo that contains coal tar or zinc pyrothione, which will slow down cell growth as well as reduce flaking. To restore oil and water balance, give the scalp, rather than the hair, a moisturizing treatment.

Dandruff Treatment for Dry Hair
1. Brush hair to remove loose dirt and flakes.
2. Heat four tablespoons of hand lotion for twenty seconds in a microwave.

3. With a clean, 1-inch paintbrush, paint warmed hand and body lotion into the hair and massage into scalp.
4. Wrap a hot, wet towel around head for twenty minutes.
5. Wash out hair with zinc pyrithione shampoo.

Keep in mind that tension will provoke an increase in dandruff problems. Since the prewedding months can be a stressful period, it is not surprising that dandruff flakes can develop at this time. To cope with unexpected flaking, add a simple aspirin rinse to your basic shampoo. Aspirin contains salicylic acid, the key ingredient in many commercial dandruff shampoos. An aspirin rinse allows you to use your favorite shampoo and conditioner while it relieves flaking.

Aspirin Antidandruff Rinse
1. Dissolve six aspirin in a cup of warm water.
2. Pour over head and work into scalp.
3. Leave on fifteen minutes.
4. Rinse thoroughly.

PROBLEM #2: HAIR LOSS

Hair loss is always troubling. But for a bride, it is wrenching. Fortunately, with the right treatment, most causes of thinning hair can be handled and reversed. The number one cause of thinning hair in the young bride would be breakage from processing and heat from hair dryers. Not infrequently, a woman with wavy or curly hair straightens the strands with a daily blast of hot air from a 1,600-watt dryer and a large paddle brush. This will indeed create a straight, smooth style—but at a price. The heat and stretching of the hair from curly to flat damages the cuticle, making the hair dull, brittle, and fragile. When enough strands break off, the loss of volume will make a woman feel she is going bald. The remedy is simple. Place a moratorium on all processing and change the way you use the hair dryer. Air-dry hair until it is damp (rather than wringing wet). Put the hair dryer heat on medium and keep the nozzle moving and at least nine inches from the head. To prevent further breakage, do the following deep, intensive conditioning every 10 days.

Preventing Problems

To avoid breakage, split ends, and hair loss, for every hour you color, straighten, wave, or blow dry your hair, commit thirty minutes to conditioning. As a general rule, the salon procedures take from forty-five to sixty minutes and blow-drying takes about fifteen minutes per session. When you do the math, it comes out to thirty to forty minutes of conditioning per week.

---

1. Combine ½ cup margarine, 2 egg yolks, 1 tablespoon cold cream. Pierce a vitamin E capsule with a pin and empty contents into mixture.
2. Paint half of the mixture onto head with a fresh, two inch paintbrush, thickly covering every strand.
3. Soak a terry-lined shower cap in hot water, wring it out, and place it on head.
4. Sit under cap for fifteen to twenty minutes.
5. Remove cap and apply rest of conditioning mixture, massaging it well into the hair.
6. Reheat cap and place on head.
7. Sit under cap for another fifteen to twenty minutes.
8. Wash out with mild shampoo and air-dry.

Daily Twenty-Minute Meditation

Effective meditation starts with creating the appropriate environment. Select a quiet room, dim the lights, and light a scented candle. Begin the meditation by focusing on your breathing. Think about each breath as you inhale and exhale. When you feel your body start to relax, direct the focus to a beautiful object in the room such as a flower or seashell. If any anxiety-provoking wedding plans pop into your thoughts, refocus on your object. Give yourself questions to mentally answer to restore your concentration on the object, such as what colors are present in it, or what the shapes of the curves and edges remind you of.

Hair loss can also occur when a diet is low in protein and calories. In our national passion for a size 4 silhouette, we can be depriving our bodies of the nutrients they need for maintenance and repair. The body shifts its concerns to the essential organs, like the heart and the brain, leaving the hair starved for food. The result is a distressing hair loss that clogs the tub and piles up on the brush. This type of hair loss is more common in vegetarians and women with eating disorders, but it can occur in anyone who eats less than five ounces of protein a day. Since this is easily met by half a roast chicken breast or a small hamburger, it is simple enough both to take in enough protein and keep weight under control.

Physical illness and emotional stress are well-documented causes of hair loss. The demands and anxieties of wedding preparation can create enough havoc to result in even more stressful hair loss. This is a self-limiting situation, and once the wedding is over, the stress ends. Unfortunately, the hair loss lags behind, and regrowth can take up to a year. Stress-provoking hair loss occurs three to four months after stress begins, and the hair regrowth cycle takes several months to kick in. To deal with stress-provoked hair loss, use stress management techniques such as meditation and exercise. These activities fool the body into changing its chemistry to reduce production of the stress hormones that are provoking problems. Research studies have demonstrated that daily meditation reduces both blood pressure and stress hormone production, helping the body feel calm and alert.

PROBLEM #3: GRAY HAIR

Gray hair is not gray, but a mixture of white hairs among the normal red, black, brown, or blond hairs. They appear as the body stops producing melanin pigment, a phenomenon that can start when a woman is still in her thirties. Stress, poor health, and even blows to the head seem to provoke graying. It is not possible to stop the development of gray hair, but it's child's play to cover it up. If there are just scattered strands around the crown and face, they can be beautifully disguised with well-placed streaks and highlights. When the gray is located around the face and hair line, it can be covered with a single-process permanent coloring that blends into natural hair tones. Although the color is permanent, it will need to be redone every six to eight weeks, as new growth appears.

Wedding Hair Coloring Options

If you color your hair, you're not alone. In the United States, one out of three women change or enhance their natural hair color. Some use hair coloring to cover gray, while other women are born-again blonds—women who were blond in childhood and want to recapture their golden hues. Then there are the fashion-forward women who are intrigued by new colors and highlighting techniques. For a bride, the months before a wedding are a time to experiment and explore a variety of colors and techniques. It is safe to experiment up to three months before the wedding. It gives you enough time to find the most flattering shade as well as to cover or repair experiments that did not work out.

The simplest colorants are temporary; they rinse out within one or two shampoos. They add a bit of depth and brightness, but certainly don't create a major change.

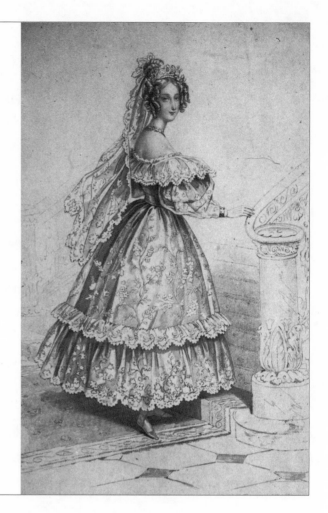

The antiroyal fervor that followed the French and American revolutions changed fashion from court extravagance to democratic simplicity. Brides used face powders enriched with a pearl essence to give their skin a luminous glow. Their pallor was enhanced by a lack of rouge and a tiny red mouth. The powered, massive hairstyles of the royals were replaced by simple smooth hair in a center part and curls over each ear. Wedding dresses were equally simple. Fashioned from sheer white muslin or organdy, they represented a romantic ideal of girlish prettiness.

Semipermanent Coloring Formulations:

Used in a color close to the hair's natural shade, they add a wonderful depth of color and shine. Although they don't last very long (ten to twelve shampoos), they are very gentle on the hair, and give an idea of how a color change would look without making a total commitment.

Tone on Tone Colorings:

Although these only allow you to deepen color and add shine, they provide long-lasting coloring without using the harsh ammonia present in most permanent tints. It is terrific for covering gray without causing dryness or damage. They need to be repeated every six to eight weeks.

Single-Process Tints:

Single-process tints offer a wide range of change that can lighten hair up to four shades. For example, if you have medium brown hair, a single process can produce a honey blond shade. Containing both peroxide to lighten and ammonia to help the color enter the hair strand, single-process tints can be drying if the hair is not conditioned regularly. Dramatic changes of color will show dark roots and will need to be retouched every three to six weeks, depending on how fast your hair grows.

Double-Process Permanent Tints:

These colorings are used to create the lightest blond shades. First, all the color is bleached out of the hair; then the desired shades are applied to the lightened hair. Unless you already are blond, this is the only way to achieve a blond shade. The color can be glorious, but double processing is the harshest form of hair coloring, needs frequent touch-ups on the roots (every three to four weeks), and can quickly lead to brittle, damaged hair. If you use double processing, you must have regular intensive conditioning at least every two weeks to restore moisture and structure to the hair.

Highlights:

Highlights are bright streaks around the face that provide sparkle without the upkeep of other types of permanent hair coloring. For this technique the hair stylist applies one to three different tones that are one to two shades lighter than natural coloring. Tiny strands of hair are coated with colorants and wrapped in foil packets to develop tone. Because there are no roots, highlighting does not need to be repeated more than every three to four months.

Lowlights:

Lowlights add depth and shine. They require the same foil wrap technique, but employ a single color that is just one shade lighter or darker than your hair's natural shade. It is a more subtle change, but still adds a beautiful richness to hair coloring. Lowlights need to be refreshed every three to four months.

COLORING YOUR HAIR FOR THE WEDDING

By the time the wedding is ten to twelve weeks away, you should have decided on the products and techniques that you will work with for the

quick tip:

Highlights Hidden View

If you highlight your hair and are planning to wear an up do at your wedding, remember that the upswept style will reveal your darker natural hair color. Sarah Classen, senior Vidal Sassoon colorist in New York, advises: "Put your hair up as you will be wearing it at your wedding and look at the back of the head in the mirror. The normally hidden lower layers of hair will be exposed and will appear much darker than the front of the hair. When you color your hair for the wedding, add highlights to the lower and back layers of the head."

ceremony. Don't use new formulations that could cause a bad reaction or result when you least want it. Color your hair no more than a week before the wedding to achieve maximum shine and tone.

Navigating the Permanent Wave

Permanents change the texture of the hair, adding volume or curl. Waving solutions use a strong alkaline formulation to permanently alter the molecules of each hair strand. There are three basic types of perms, and all are available in both beauty salons and in home kits. Conventional waves use ammonium thioglycolate to alter hair structure. Mild formulations add body and volume, while higher concentrations produce curls and waves. Acid waves, which are less alkaline, tend to be less damaging to the hair and produce a softer curl. Available only in beauty salons and beauty supply companies, they can be used more safely with color treated, thin, or fragile hair. Soft waves, the gentlest form of perm, use bisulfide formulations, and they are the most frequently used product in home perm kits and have less of a chance of producing frizz or breakage.

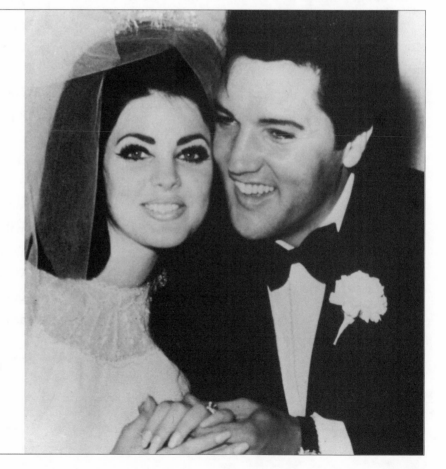

CLOSE-UP:
Priscilla Presley
....

Priscilla *Beaulieu was a beautiful fourteen-year-old with dark brown hair when she met Elvis Presley. At her wedding to the King, her hair had been dyed to match his own inky black color.*

Although they last only two to three months, they are a good choice if you color-treat your hair.

By reading the information in a home kit, you will be able to learn if the perm formulation is conventional acid or soft perm. In a salon, you won't see the product until it's on your hair. So it's important that you meet with your stylist to discuss the type of perm that will give you the results you want. The permanent wave puts a strain on the hair, leaving it vulnerable to dryness and breakage. It should be treated with low-pH shampoos, and frequent deep conditioning treatments as described on page 43. Avoid creme rinse conditioners, which soften the hair strand.

Reverse Perms: Straightening the Hair

For every woman who turns to a perm for body or curls, there's another who turns to straightening to relax coarse or curly hair. Usually a lye formulation, a straightener is combed through the damp hair to soften and straighten each strand. The effects are permanent, but as new hair grows in, curls and coarse texture will return at the roots. Most stylists recommend repeating straightening only two—at the most, three—times a year. If you want straight hair for your wedding, try straightening at least six months before the wedding. If you like the effect, repeat the procedure one month before the wedding. When used together, hair coloring and straightening can cause problems if not handled properly. If you want to relax the hair, hair coloring should use the gentlest products, like semipermanent or single-process, in a color close to your own hair shade. Avoid dramatic color changes that require frequent touch-ups and double-processing that strips color from the hair shaft. Always wait two to three weeks between coloring and relaxing the hair. Relaxed hair needs a regular program of low pH shampoos and conditioners, as described for colored or waved hair.

As you did with skin care products, create a box for wedding-day hair care. When you find shampoo you like, buy a fresh bottle, label it, and put it away. This way you are sure to have everything you need on your wedding day, and it's one less thing to worry about.

Hair Care Products

* Shampoo for specific hair type
* Creme rinse
* Instant conditioner
* Deep conditioner
* Lemon juice
* Wide tooth comb
* Hair pins
* Bobby pins
* Styling clips
* Brush
* Hair spray
* Thermal hair spray

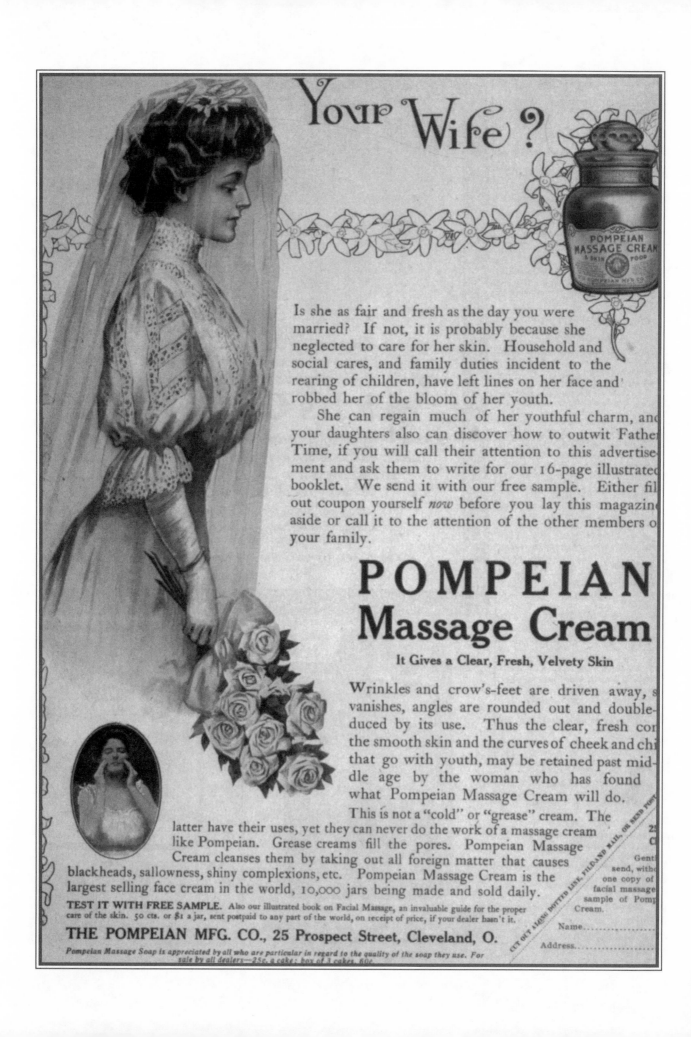

Your Wife?

Is she as fair and fresh as the day you were married? If not, it is probably because she neglected to care for her skin. Household and social cares, and family duties incident to the rearing of children, have left lines on her face and robbed her of the bloom of her youth.

She can regain much of her youthful charm, and your daughters also can discover how to outwit Father Time, if you will call their attention to this advertisement and ask them to write for our 16-page illustrated booklet. We send it with our free sample. Either fill out coupon yourself *now* before you lay this magazine aside or call it to the attention of the other members of your family.

POMPEIAN
Massage Cream

It Gives a Clear, Fresh, Velvety Skin

Wrinkles and crow's-feet are driven away, s vanishes, angles are rounded out and double-duced by its use. Thus the clear, fresh co the smooth skin and the curves of cheek and chi that go with youth, may be retained past mid-dle age by the woman who has found what Pompeian Massage Cream will do.

This is not a "cold" or "grease" cream. The latter have their uses, yet they can never do the work of a massage cream like Pompeian. Grease creams fill the pores. Pompeian Massage Cream cleanses them by taking out all foreign matter that causes blackheads, sallowness, shiny complexions, etc. Pompeian Massage Cream is the largest selling face cream in the world, 10,000 jars being made and sold daily.

TEST IT WITH FREE SAMPLE. Also our illustrated book on Facial Massage, an invaluable guide for the proper care of the skin. 50 cts. or $1 a jar, sent postpaid to any part of the world, on receipt of price, if your dealer hasn't it.

THE POMPEIAN MFG. CO., 25 Prospect Street, Cleveland, O.

Pompeian Massage Soap is appreciated by all who are particular in regard to the quality of the soap they use. For sale by all dealers—25c. a cake; box of 3 cakes, 60c.

POMPEIAN MASSAGE CREAM & SKIN FOOD POMPEIAN MFG CO

CUT OUT ALONG DOTTED LINE, FILL AND MAIL, OR SEND POST

Gent send, witho one copy of facial massage sample of Pomp Cream.

Name......................
Address...................

CHAPTER FOUR

The Bridal Body

goals:
....

* **To tone and define body silhouette**
* **To establish long-term healthy eating habits**

It has been said that if a female feels comfortable about her body in a bathing suit, she's probably no more than six years old. We tend to focus on what we perceive as negatives. We wish we were taller, thinner, our legs longer, our arms firmer. When we become engaged, one of the first thoughts that enters our minds is, "I've got to go on a diet."

First, take a deep breath. Your fiancé has chosen to spend his life with you just the way you are. Whether or not you lose ten pounds is not going to make the difference in his love for you or even in the success of your wedding. Rest assured that whatever your body's strengths and weaknesses, you will be able to find a dress that will be beautiful and flattering.

That said, if you are carrying some extra pounds, an upcoming wedding can be one of the strongest motivators that you will ever experience. Excess weight is never healthy at any age. According to Celle Lalli, long-time editor in chief of *Modern Bride,* the prewedding months provide a wonderful opportunity to get your body in great shape. "A bridal diet, skin care, and exercise program will not only result in a glorious wedding look, it can establish a healthy lifestyle for the years to come," she advised.

Diet for a Beautiful Bride

However well-motivated you may be, it is important to set realistic goals. If you have always struggled with a weight problem, it is probably not possible to lose enough weight prior to your wedding to radically change your basic shape. Traditionally, the most you can expect to lose is two pounds per week, even if you adhere to a rigorous diet and exercise plan. The prewedding months are a hectic and social time, with parties, lunches, and dinners with friends and family. Even if you would like to take off more weight, it is best to plan on losing a maximum of about ten to fifteen pounds. This weight loss will not change the style of dress that flatters your body shape— this is pretty much determined by your height and bone structure—but you will look trimmer and feel better in your gown.

If you are committed to losing weight, inform the bridal consultant where you buy your dress that you are on a serious diet. Depending on the style of the dress, the bridal salon may order the dress one size smaller than your current measurements would indicate.

To be successful in your weight loss goals, you need a plan that combines diet and walking with weight training to shape and tone. The plan must be easy to follow at work, at home, and when eating out with friends and family. This is not a time for a diet that requires special meals and time-intensive exercises.

MEASURE EVERYTHING

The diet that follows is a portion-control diet that carefully watches all nutritional components. It is sugar-free and low in salt, fat, calories, and cholesterol. It is a healthy diet that meets the minimum daily requirements of all nutrients, and it can be followed so that it doesn't restrict you socially. The meals can be easily prepared at home and are available in restaurants from the simplest coffee shop to the most elaborate gourmet restaurant.

The key to following this diet is quantity control. You have to carefully measure each portion. When you are eating out, gauge the size of the portion carefully. For example, the recommended portion of meat is two to three ounces per serving, which is about the size of a small hamburger or turkey burger in a restaurant. But if you order steak or chicken, you will usually get eight ounces of beef, or half a chicken, which is more than twice the portion that you should be consuming at each meal. You can follow the menu choices without deviation, but if you exceed portion size, the weight will not come off.

Proteins are limited to five to six ounces of fish, veal, chicken, or turkey per day. Restrict eggs to just the whites (three per serving) for low fat omelettes. Red meat should be eaten no more than once per week for either lunch or dinner. All proteins can be roasted, broiled, poached, or grilled, but not fried or braised.

There are five portions of carbohydrates per day, a portion being a half cup of cooked rice, corn, potatoes, cereal, or pasta or one slice of bread. The first time that you measure out pasta or rice, you probably will be surprised how small it is compared to the serving size usually offered in restaurants.

Fats are limited to one tablespoon a day of olive oil, margarine, mayonnaise, or salad dressing. If you wish, you can use two tablespoons of fat-free margarine, mayonnaise, or salad dressing instead. Measure these quantities carefully. These incidental fats can make or break your diet.

Fresh green vegetables can be eaten in any quantity and should be eaten at least two or three times a day. This isn't nearly as much as it sounds. A serving of tomatoes can be as little as two slices, and lettuce is a few crisp leaves. You can eat more, but you don't have to force yourself. Vegetables can be eaten raw or cooked without oil or margarine.

Fruits are limited to two servings per day. The fruit should be fresh rather than canned or cooked. The menus use fruits that are available year-round in most regions, but you should take advantage of seasonal products in your area.

Milk products are important for calcium to provide strength for your nails and for your bones. You should have two 1-cup servings of fat-free milk or yogurt per day. Hard cheese is not a good source of calcium because it is so high in fat and cottage cheese is surprisingly high in calories and sugars. For a special treat, you can have half a cup of sugar-free, fat-free frozen dessert instead of yogurt three times a week. To avoid weight plateaus, make sure that you use fat-free milk in your tea or coffee.

In addition to the basic diet program, you must include at least a brisk twenty- to thirty-minute walk every single day. This is to stimulate your metabolism, and it can be easily worked into even the busiest schedule by simply walking to or from work, or, if you take public transportation, you can stop a mile from your home or office and walk the extra way. If you drive, try parking in a lot about a half a mile to a mile from your office.

This diet will chisel ten to fifteen pounds of real—not water—weight off almost everyone, a weight loss that will make a nice change in the way your gown fits.

This seven-day meal plan is designed to demonstrate how the diet works. You can substitute any fruit, vegetable, or fish for the listed item in a menu. You can also switch around a lunch or dinner for a different day. Dishes designated with a star indicate that a recipe is provided.

Day One

BREAKFAST:

½ cup low-sugar cereal, for example, Corn Flakes, Special K, Cheerios, Wheat Chex, Puffed Wheat, or Puffed Rice, with ½ cup of skim milk

SNACK:

½ grapefruit

LUNCH:

A 3-ounce turkey burger

2 slices tomato

1 onion ring

2 leaves lettuce

2 slices of whole wheat toast

Decaffeinated coffee or tea

SNACK:

1 slice of melon

DINNER:

3 ounces roast chicken★

1 cup cooked broccoli

½ cup brown rice

1 cup fat-free, sugar-free yogurt

Day Two

BREAKFAST:

2 slices sourdough toast

2 slices tomato

1 tablespoon light cream cheese

SNACK:

½ grapefruit

LUNCH:

2 ounces water-packed tuna

2 teaspoons fat-free mayonnaise

2 slices of whole wheat bread

2 leaves lettuce

2 slices tomato

SNACK:

1 apple

DINNER:

3 ounces swordfish★

2 tablespoons salsa★

3 tiny steamed new potatoes

1 sliced cucumber, sprinkled with dill

Day Three

BREAKFAST:

Egg-white omelette with mushrooms

2 slices whole wheat toast

SNACK:

½ cup grapes

LUNCH:

Green salad with 1 tablespoon fat-free dressing

2 ounces roast turkey

2 slices sourdough toast

SNACK:

1 orange

DINNER:

2 ounces roast turkey breast★

½ cup roast carrots and potatoes★

½ cup broccoli

If the Diet Isn't Working

There could be two reasons why pounds refuse to budge. It could simply be that a bride is skimping on the length and intensity of exercises. Frequently weight plateaus can result when fat intake exceeds recommended portions. It is all too easy to add extra fat and calories. An extra tablespoon of salad dressing, some margarine on cooked vegetables, or a drizzle of olive oil on broiled fish, and you've added 300 calories per day. Focus your attention on the fat, and the weight should start to drift down.

Day Four

BREAKFAST:

½ cup oatmeal

½ cup skim milk

SNACK:

½ grapefruit

LUNCH:

3 ounces low-fat tuna salad★

2 slices whole wheat bread

SNACK:

1 slice melon

DINNER:

3 ounces Cajun shrimp★

2 cups green salad with 1–2 tablespoons fat-free Italian dressing

1 slice garlic bread

½ cup sugar-free Jell-O

Day Five

BREAKFAST:

1 toasted pita

2 teaspoons sugar-free jam

SNACK:

1 cup strawberries

LUNCH:

Low-fat grilled cheese and tomato sandwich

Salad with 1–2 tablespoons fat-free Russian dressing

SNACK:

½ grapefruit

DINNER:

½ breast of oven-fried chicken★

1 cup steamed green beans

½ ear corn

½ cup coleslaw★

Day Six

BREAKFAST:

½ cup low-sugar, low-fat cold cereal

½ cup fat-free milk

SNACK:

1 orange

LUNCH:

Sliced turkey sandwich on whole wheat bread with 2 ounces of meat and 2 tablespoons Russian dressing

½ cup of coleslaw★

SNACK:

1 apple

DINNER:

3–4 ounces baked salmon★

½ cup brown rice

½ cup steamed snow peas

Day Seven

BREAKFAST:

2 slices bridal french toast

1–2 tablespoons sugar-free syrup

SNACK:

½ grapefruit

LUNCH:

1 cup chicken soup

1 cup green salad with 1 tablespoon fat-free dressing

1 cup sugar-free Jell-O

SNACK:

1 cup sliced strawberries

DINNER:

5 ounces veal chop★

½ cup baby green beans

½ cup mashed potatoes

½ cup sliced cucumbers

Dress for the Body You Have

If you are starting out to look for a dress, and you are planning to take off some pounds, don't buy a dress in a style that requires a different body shape than the one you have. For example, if you have a large bust, don't buy a dress with a round, high neck that really needs a tall, thin, angular frame to look beautiful. You are not going to change your body type that much with a ten- or fifteen-pound weight loss to make that dress work for you. Choose the dress that is inherently flattering to your basic form. Perhaps you can even order it in a size smaller than you are taking now, with the thought that it is going to be custom-tailored. It is far better to have a dress beautifully cut for your body than to force your body into wearing a dress that just generally won't work for you.

Recipes

Roast Chicken

1   whole chicken (3–4 pounds)
1   teaspoon meat tenderizer
1   teaspoon kosher salt
¼   teaspoon black pepper
        Juice of 1 lemon (keep the rinds)
2   scallions, diced

1. Preheat oven to 450°F.
2. Wash chicken under cool running water.
3. Slip hand under skin to loosen it.
4. Combine meat tenderizer, salt, pepper, and lemon juice and spoon under chicken skin.
5. Place chicken in plastic bag, seal, and refrigerate for 2 hours.
6. Remove chicken from plastic bag. Tuck in wings and tie legs together with cotton twine.
7. Stuff chicken with lemon rinds and scallions.
8. Place chicken in roasting pan that has been sprayed with vegetable oil spray.
9. Roast chicken at 450°F for 1 hour.

Swordfish with Salsa

8   ounces swordfish
        Salt and pepper to taste
1   teaspoon olive oil

1. Preheat oven to 400°F.
2. Season fish with salt and pepper.
3. Heat olive oil in sauté pan.
4. Brown swordfish on both sides, about 3 minutes per side.
5. Place in 8 × 12" baking dish and bake in oven for 10 minutes.
6. Serve with salsa.

Salsa

2	tomatoes, chopped
1	tablespoon chopped red onion
1	clove of garlic, chopped
½	cup green pepper, chopped
1	tablespoon parsley, finely chopped
1	tablespoon lemon juice
1	jalapeño pepper, seeded and chopped

1. Combine all ingredients and chill in refrigerator for several hours.

Roast Turkey Breast with Carrots and Potatoes

1	cup small white onions
4	carrots, cut into 2-inch pieces
1	tablespoon fresh rosemary
½	turkey breast (3–4 pounds)
12	small new potatoes
½	teaspoon black pepper to taste
1	tablespoon olive oil

1. Preheat oven to 375°F.
2. Spray tin foil–lined 9 × 12" roasting pan with vegetable oil spray.
3. Place half the onions and carrots plus 1 teaspoon rosemary in the pan.
4. Lay turkey on vegetables.
5. Position rest of vegetables around turkey.
6. Sprinkle remaining rosemary, ½ teaspoon black pepper, and olive oil over turkey and vegetables.
7. Roast for 1 hour or until meat thermometer registers 170°F.

Low-fat Tuna Salad

    1   6-ounce can water-packed tuna
    1   tablespoon chopped fresh dill
    1   tablespoon chopped red onion
    1   tablespoon grated carrot
    1   tablespoon chopped celery
    1   tablespoon fat-free mayonnaise
    1   tablespoon plain fat-free yogurt
    1   teaspoon lemon juice
  ¼   teaspoon black pepper
Whole wheat bread or lettuce, for garnish

1. Mix tuna, dill, red onion, carrot, and celery in a bowl.
2. Combine mayonnaise, yogurt, black pepper, and lemon juice in a small bowl.
3. Mix seasoned mayonnaise with tuna and vegetables.
4. Serve on whole wheat bread or bed of lettuce.

Hot Cajun Shrimp Salad

  2   teaspoons olive oil
  2   teaspoons Cajun seasoning
  ½   pound raw medium shrimp, shelled and deveined
  1   lemon quarter
  3   cups mixed greens

1. Combine olive oil and Cajun seasoning and toss with shrimp.
2. Grill shrimp in nonstick pan for 3–5 minutes.
3. Squeeze lemon juice over shrimp.
4. Pour hot shrimp on mixed greens and serve.

Oven-Fried Chicken

½   cup cornflakes, crushed

½   teaspoon each of dry mustard, paprika, onion powder, and black
     pepper

1   pound chicken pieces, skinned

2   egg whites, beaten

1. Preheat oven to 350°F.
2. Mix cornflakes and seasonings in a small bowl.
3. Dip chicken in egg whites and dredge in cornflakes mixture.
4. Spray foil-covered baking sheet with vegetable oil spray.
5. Lay chicken pieces on baking sheet and spray chicken with
   vegetable oil spray.
6. Bake for 30 minutes, turning pieces over once.

Coleslaw

½   head cabbage, finely shredded

1   large carrot, grated

2   teaspoons kosher salt

2   tablespoons thinly sliced onion

¼   cup fat-free mayonnaise

¼   cup plain fat-free yogurt

1   tablespoon parsley, finely chopped

1. Toss cabbage and grated carrot with salt and let stand at room
   temperature for 2 hours in a colander.
2. Dump cabbage and carrot into cold water rinse.
3. Put vegetables back into colander, pressing them down to drain.
4. Pat dry with paper towels.
5. Put cabbage and carrots into a bowl. Add onion, mayonnaise, and
   yogurt to coat.
6. Sprinkle with parsley.
7. Refrigerate 1 hour before serving.

Every Bride Is
Beautiful

Baked Salmon Fillet

½   pound salmon fillet
4   tablespoons plain fat-free yogurt
2   teaspoons capers
1   teaspoon paprika

1. Preheat oven to 400°F. Spray tin foil–covered pan with vegetable oil spray.
2. Cut salmon into 2 portions.
3. Place salmon in pan, and cover each piece with 2 tablespoons yogurt.
4. Sprinkle each piece with 1 teaspoon capers and dust with paprika.
5. Bake 20 minutes at 400°F.

Veal Chops with Mushrooms

1   teaspoon olive oil
2   loin veal chops (about 1 pound)
Salt and pepper to taste
½   pound sliced mushrooms
1   lemon quarter

1. Preheat oven to 400°F.
2. Heat olive oil in medium-size frying pan.
3. Brown veal chops on each side about 3 minutes per side. Remove chops and place in shallow baking dish.
4. Bake in 9 × 12" pan for 10 minutes at 400°F.
5. While chops are baking, sauté mushrooms in nonstick pan.
6. Season mushrooms with salt and pepper and lemon juice.
7. Remove veal chops from oven; arrange them on a plate and cover with mushrooms.

Body Shaping 101

To sculpt body shape and improve tone, a diet and walking program must be combined with a series of body-contouring exercises that utilize weight training.

Dimples and ripples on a healthy baby are adorable, but they seem to lose their charm on an adult body. These shape irregularities are actually a sign of a loss of muscle strength and volume. When you work out with weights, you make tiny tears in the muscle. As these tears heal, the muscle builds up in volume and strength. Don't be afraid that you will develop the large, bulging muscles of a bodybuilder. What you will do is create is a trimmer and more beautiful silhouette.

BEAUTIFUL ARMS

We can usually hide loss of tone under jackets, blouses, and sweaters, but wedding gowns reveal parts of the body usually seen only by your lover or your mother. The body part that seems to be a bride's number one concern is usually her upper arms. The sleeveless, short-sleeve, off-shoulder, or slip dresses all seem to magnify less-than-perfect shapes.

There are two sets of muscles in the upper arms: the triceps, on the back of the upper arm, and the biceps, a large muscle mass at the front of the arm. If either group of muscles is weak and small, the arm looks plump and flabby.

Bridal Exercise #1:
Biceps

1. Lie on your back and hold a 3-pound dumbbell straight up in the air with your hands.
2. Bend elbows slowly toward your chest.
3. Repeat 10 times with each arm.

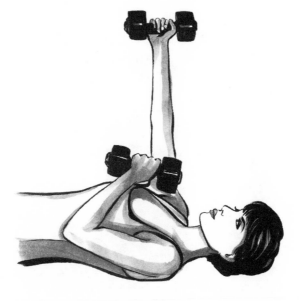

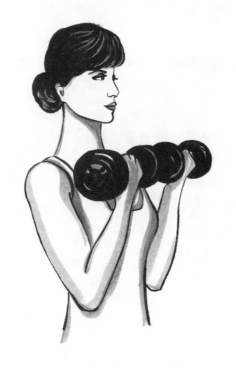

Bridal Exercise #2:
Triceps

1. Stand straight with a 3-pound dumbbell in each hand.
2. Slowly swing your arms up to chest level with palms toward your face.
3. Repeat 10 times.

A TRIMMER WAISTLINE

The muscles along the rib cage produce a flat, smooth waistline that enhances the bodice of any style of wedding gown. Diet can remove pounds, but exercise creates the line most brides want.

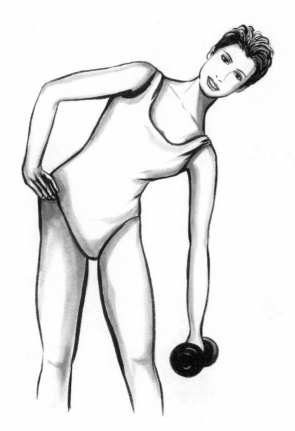

Bridal Exercise #3

1. Stand with arms at side, shoulders back, feet square with your shoulders.
2. Hold a 3-pound dumbbell in your left hand and bend slowly down the left side.
3. Repeat 10 times.
4. Switch dumbbell to right hand and bend waist and shoulders to right side.

TONING THE OTHER CHEEKS

During the bridal ceremony, much of the time the bride has her back to the wedding guests. If there was ever a time to tone and lift the buttocks, this would be it.

Bridal Exercise #4

1. Lie on the floor with knees bent and feet flat on the floor.
2. Lift pelvis and tighten the buttocks, keeping your back straight.
3. Press thighs together and hold for 10 seconds.
4. Repeat 10 times.
5. With legs apart, lift pelvis, keeping feet flat.
6. Repeat 10 times.

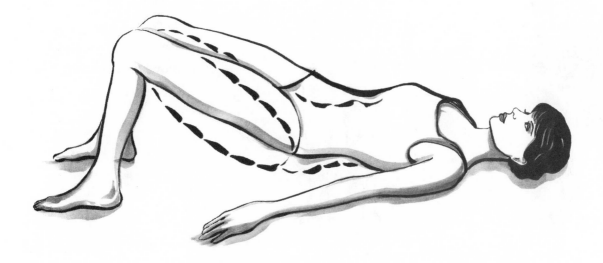

The Truth About Spot Reducing

Exercise cannot reduce fat in specific areas. True weight loss is only possible with a diet that reduces calories and an exercise program that encourages the body to burn calories. Exercising selected muscles with weights builds muscle mass and tones the body, creating a firmer, more attractive silhouette, but it does not actually eliminate weight in any one spot.

Every Bride Is Beautiful

A BEAUTIFUL BACK

Strong back muscles promote good posture and a graceful gait, essential for a beautiful walk down the aisle, as well as a graceful walk for the rest of your life.

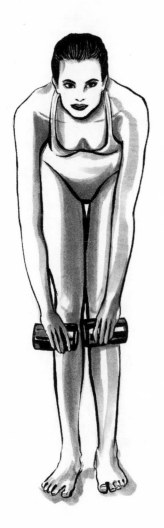 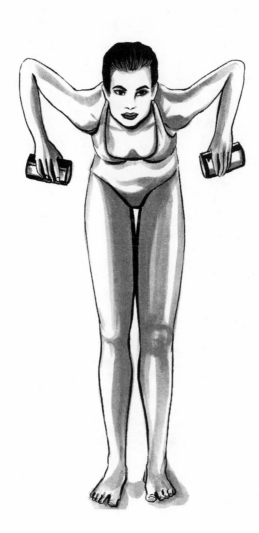

Bridal Exercise #5

1. Stand straight with 3-pound dumbbells in each hand.
2. Bend over at the waist and, with back flat and arms hanging down, pull hands up with elbows out to the sides.
3. Pause for a count of 5.
4. Slowly bring hands down.
5. Repeat 10 times.

Care of Body Skin

In addition to concern about shape and size, the body-baring lines of a wedding gown make you all too aware of the usually covered skin on your body. When it comes to skin care, we tend to lavish time and attention on the face. In general, we slide legs into jeans, pull on a sweater, and ignore the rest of the body. The first time a bride tries on a wedding gown, she suddenly becomes aware of the other 95 percent of her skin. The job of many wedding gowns is to show skin, with low necklines and sleeveless styles. The skin on the shoulders, arms, and neck is suddenly unveiled. When you sit down to try on white satin wedding sandals, you realize that you are suddenly showing your legs and heels, while honeymoon-bound swimwear now reveals your bottom and thighs. To give the rest of your body the care it needs, you need a program of cleansing, protection, and moisturizing.

SOAPS

To create smooth, clear body skin, you need to combine thorough cleansing with gentle exfoliation. The skin should be cleaned with a moisturizing soap and a smooth loofah or sponge. Soap will clean the body of dirt and oil, but a slightly abrasive brush or sponge is essential to stimulate circulation and to remove dry, dulling skin cells that cling to the surface. The first time you do this, you will notice a gentle tingle and a feeling of freshness. To produce and maintain results, body cleansing and exfoliation should be done every day. The choice of soap depends on your skin needs.

There are basically three different kinds of formulations: traditional bar soaps, moisturizing, creamy, liquid cleansers, and gel cleansers. Each can be modified, depending on what other ingredients they contain.

Super-fatted Soaps:
These soaps contain extra amounts of oil and are good for normal or slightly dry skin. The increased fat and oil content prevents the soap from stripping off all the moisture. If you have very oily or acne-prone skin on your face, even if your body skin is dry, this is probably not a good choice.

Castile Soaps:
Castile soaps have olive oil as their main fat. They are slightly richer than the basic soap and often somewhat more expensive. Excellent for drier skins.

Transparent Soaps:
Originally for dry skin, these soaps are made with little or no alcohol and have been modified for all types of skin textures. They do an excellent job of cleansing, are very mild, and are available in both liquid and bar form.

Deodorant Soaps:
These soaps contain antibacterial chemicals that kill the bacteria normally present on the skin that lead to body odor. Without the bacteria, the body

Queen Victoria

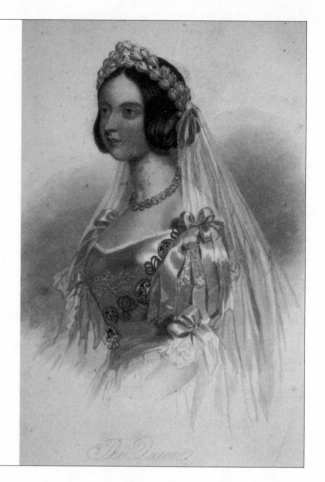

In the first half of the nineteenth century, all of England was enchanted with the 1840 marriage of the beautiful young Queen Victoria to her beloved Prince Albert. Her wedding ensemble was a radical change from the gold and jeweled bridal clothing worn for centuries for royal weddings. Her gown of white silk was decorated with swags of lace and studded with tiny silk flowers. On her head she wore a wreath of orange blossoms (a symbol of fertility) instead of a crown. Around her face was draped a long flowing lace veil crafted from forty yards of handmade Honiton lace. The wedding of Queen Victoria established white as the color for the wedding gown and created bridal styles and standards that we still follow today.

skin stays fresher longer. Antibacterial soaps also kill bacteria, but their purpose is to protect against contamination that can lead to illness, such as food-borne and respiratory illnesses, colds and flu.

Floating Soaps:

These soaps are manufactured with extra water and air trapped inside them. They don't have any special properties for your skin, but you won't lose a bar at the bottom of the tub.

Oatmeal Soaps:

Oatmeal soaps are an interesting formulation because they not only absorb oil and dirt, but also soothe the skin. It often is one of the least irritating soaps and is good for sensitive skins.

Detergent Soaps:

These soaps may conjure up an image of harsh chemicals, but it's actually easier for cosmetic chemists to make a detergent soap less alkaline, dehydrating, and irritating. They are often used in sensitive-skin formulations.

Acne Soaps:

These are used by people with acne- or oily-prone skin, and they are best used for the face. If you also have breakout problems on your chest and back, this is also a good soap to use in these areas, but it is probably too drying to use on the rest of the body.

Bath Soap:

This simply refers to the size of the bar; it's usually larger than the hand soap used at the sink.

Cocoa Butter Soaps:

These soaps use cocoa butter as the main fat ingredient; they are favorites of people with dry skin.

Aloe Soaps:

Aloe has a soothing and healing effect on the skin, and it is felt that the aloe decreases the harshness and the alkalinity of many soaps.

The choice of bar or gel is a personal one. However, gel cleansers are usually better for normal skin, while moisturizing cleansers are better for drier skins. If you have sensitive skin, you will probably do well with products that have little or no fragrance, since about half of all allergic reactions to cosmetics are caused by the fragrance.

Soap should be applied to an abrasive mitt such as a sponge or loofah and stroked on the body. The improvement in circulation from the loofah not only makes the skin softer, but may be helpful in reducing deposits of a lumpy fat called cellulite. It has been suggested that scrubbing with a sponge helps break down the fatty pockets of this lumpy fat.

MOISTURIZERS

While we all have different skin textures on our face, the skin of most bodies tends to become dry. At best, we have a naturally inadequate moisturizing system. Most of the oil glands are located on the face and back. The plan is for the oil to work its way across the rest of the body. As every woman who has applied cases of lotion to dry elbows and flaky legs knows, our natural moisturizing system leaves a lot to be desired. Dry skin looks dull and feels itchy. One of the best ways to getting a handle on the problem is to choose the right moisturizer. The base of all creams and lotions is a mixture of wax, water, and oil. Massaged into the skin, it forms a protective shield on the surface of the skin to trap skin-softening moisture. This works well as long as the cream remains on the skin; once it wears away, the dryness returns. What gives hand and body lotions longer-lasting impact are natural moisturizing elements that attract and hold water in the skin.

The newest and one of the most popular ingredients in moisturizers today are the alpha-hydroxy acids. These natural compounds are derived from fruits and dairy products such as apples, sugar cane, and milk. Also known as fruit acids, they soften the skin by taking off the top dead layer of skin cells and encouraging the skin to hold water. Their softening impact will last hours after any trace of the moisturizer has disappeared.

Hyaluronic acid is a substance naturally found in the skin whose job is to hold moisture. As we grow older, our level of hyaluronic acid goes down; moisturizers that contain this element encourage the skin to stay softer. One of the most interesting ingredients you might find in a moisturizer are phospholipid, or lipids, which actually form a netting on the surface of the skin and trap water to soften and soothe the skin. We naturally have phospholipid in our skin; this is another element that decreases as we get older. Lecithin, which is found in egg yolks, is one of the most commonly used lipids and is an excellent addition to a daily hand and body cream.

The impact of a moisturizer is also related to the type of oil that it contains. Vegetable oils, such as corn, safflower, and olive oils, are excellent in our diet, and they make a decent moisturizer. Animal fats such as lanolin are closest to our natural skin oils, and they do a very good job of holding in moisture. Some people may be sensitive to lanolin and would then best choose a vegetable oil. There are some exotic, expensive oils, such as mink oil or turtle oil, that are probably used in such small amounts in a product that they have no impact.

You should really stay away from products heavily based on mineral oil. Mineral oil products are not good for the face, but do a good job on the body. Mineral oils such as petroleum jelly create a moisturizing shield on the skin surface, but if you have a tendency to break out, it can cause problems. Even if you don't put it on your face, it can be on your hands, and when you touch your face it may provoke breakouts on oily or acne-prone skin. In these cases you should reserve mineral oil products for your feet and elbows and keep them away from your face, neck, and chest.

SUN PROTECTION

Sunscreens are a wonderful addition to daytime hand and body creams. A good sunscreen not only helps to prevent your skin's aging, but also blocks the development of freckles and discolorations. The low-necked, backless and sleeveless wedding gowns call for clear, smooth, unblemished skin, and the use of a sunscreen for three to four months prior to a wedding will reduce existing brown spots and prevent formation of new ones. Getting into the habit of using a fortified moisturizer not only results in a clear, smooth wedding complexion, but also will reduce signs of aging for years to come.

BATH OR SHOWER?

While both do an excellent job of cleansing, there are benefits and drawbacks to both baths and showers. A long soak in a relaxing bath can relieve prewedding stress, reduce muscle ache, and soften the skin. Keep in mind, however, that sitting in a hot bath for more than fifteen to twenty minutes can actually rob the skin of essential oils and increase dryness. A quick shower is efficient and refreshing, but may not give you the time to give your skin the attention it deserves. To make the most of your shower, use exfoliators with your soap. The best solution for many women is to use showers for daily care, reserving one night a week for a luxurious, long bath.

The Complete Shower

1. Turn on your shower to warm up and moisturize the bathroom. Before you step in, make sure you have all you need: shampoo, conditioner, back brush, bath soap or gel, facial cleanser, loofah mitt, razor (if shaving), towels, wide tooth comb.
2. Wet entire body, then apply soap to exfoliator and, starting at your neck, gently buff the skin. As you move downward, keep an even, circular motion to cleanse skin as you stimulate circulation and remove dry skin.
3. Switch to a bath brush to cleanse skin over back and shoulders. Go all the way down to the feet, but don't wash the soles with the soap to avoid falling on the slippery floor.

A warm, scented bath cleanses the body, softens the skin, relieves muscle aches, and restores the spirit. For best results, keep water temperature between 97°F and 99°F, since overhot bath water can put a strain on the heart and dry out the skin. Vary your bathing experience by adding special ingredients:

* A handful of bath crystals soften hard water
* ½ cup of cornstarch or oatmeal can soothe irritated or sunburned skin
* Bath oils relieve dry, itchy skin
* A few drops of an essential oil such as almond oil can relax the mind as well as the body
* Milk and milk products such as yogurt, buttermilk, or powered milk contain lactic acid, which smoothes away dead, dry skin.

4. Stand under a stream of shower to rinse thoroughly. Wash and condition hair according to directions and the suggestions in chapter 3.
5. If you shave your legs, do it now. The warm water and exfoliation will soften the hairs and prevent ingrown hairs.
6. When you get out of the shower, sit down and massage your feet with a soapy loofah. Concentrate on the rough areas at the sides and back of the heels. Remove soap with a warm, wet washcloth.
7. Dry feet and body thoroughly. Then while skin is slightly damp, apply hand and body lotion, starting at the neck.

The Perfect Bath

1. Take the phone off the hook, put on your favorite CD or tape, and light two fat bayberry candles.
2. Fill the tub with comfortably warm water, add a bath enrichment such as almond oil or one of the bath recipes that follow.
3. Turn out the lights and step into the tub.
4. Lay back against the bath pillow and visualize that you are in a place that you love.
5. After fifteen minutes, apply cleanser to a loofah or bath sponge and massage your entire body.
6. Stand up and rinse under a shower.
7. Step out of the tub, turn on the light, and blow out the candles.
7. Towel-dry the skin and, while it is still slightly damp, apply body lotion.

Milk Bath

Combine 1 cup buttermilk and 1 tablespoon peach kernel oil and pour into warm bath.

Honey Spice Bath

Combine 1 cup whole milk yogurt, 1 tablespoon honey, ¼ teaspoon ground cinnamon, and one pinch of ground cloves and pour into warm bath.

Herbal Infusion Bath

Combine 2 tablespoons of dried rosemary, 1 tablespoon dried mint, and 1 tablespoon dried thyme with 1 cup boiling water. Steep herbs for 30 minutes, strain and discard herbs, saving the herbal-scented infusion. Pour the entire cup into warm bath.

> ### Bridal Bath Product Shopping List
>
> * Bath pillow
> * Loofah
> * Body cleanser
> * Body lotion
> * Bayberry candles
> * Favorite CD or tape
> * Bath oil
> * Oatmeal
> * Powdered milk
> * Bath crystals
> * Thick, large terry towels

THE DELICATE TRUTH ABOUT BATH POWDER

Bath powder is one of the oldest known toiletries. In the days before thick, thirsty terry cloth towels, women used only thin cloths to dry their bodies after a bath. Because they were particularly ineffective, they left the body soggy. Women used talc to absorb remaining moisture. It leaves a luxurious, soft texture to the skin, as it whitens tones. Unfortunately, because body powder is so good at absorbing moisture, it can increase skin dryness. If you love to use fragrant body powder, reserve it for areas where moisture tends to accumulate, such as inner thighs and under the arms, rather than on the drier areas, such as shoulders and legs.

THE HAIR WE DON'T WANT

We all want a full, thick head of hair on our head. But when the hair production starts to drift south to our faces and bodies, it becomes a major nuisance. The skin-revealing wedding styles and honeymoon bikinis motivate a bride to find the best way to eliminate unwanted hair growth. Options range from practically free to terribly expensive, from painless to toe-curling.

Every Bride Is Beautiful

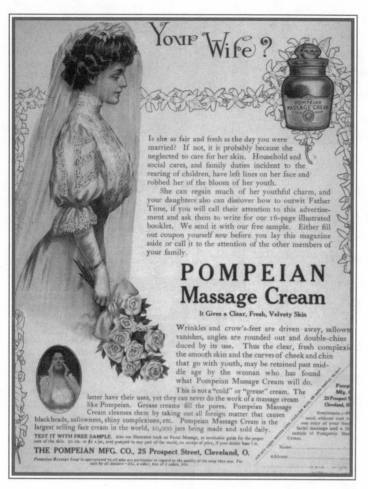

Shaving with a razor cuts off the hair at the skin level. For the legs and underarms, it does an adequate, albeit temporary, job of hair removal. Fast, simple and inexpensive, you will get smoother results if you use a shaving gel to soften hairs as you shave.

Chemical depilatories contain thioglycolic acid, which weakens hairs so they break off slightly below the skin surface. Lasting a bit longer than shaving, they are used for legs, underarms, the upper lip and chin. Women are often put off by the smell—think rotten eggs—while others may develop an itchy red skin reaction. If you've never used depilatories before, don't try it less than a month before the wedding.

Waxing spreads hot wax on the skin; it is allowed to cool slightly, then is pulled off with a smooth, even motion. Wax takes off the hair and part of the root, but not the hair bulb. Because it takes out the entire hair, it takes three to six weeks to grow back. Although this is not considered a permanent form of hair removal, repeated waxings create enough damage at the hair bulb that regrowth decreases. The bad news: It hurts, even when done by skilled professionals (and it should only be done by professionals). Waxing feels exactly like what it is: Yanking hair out by its roots. Despite discomfort, its smooth, long-lasting results make waxing one of the most popular forms of hair removal.

To relieve discomfort, take aspirin or an ibuprofen after waxing the legs and thighs. If you regularly smooth skin with a loofah or scrub mitt, you will avoid ingrown hairs. Don't wait until the wedding to try waxing for the first time. Some skin develops small red bumps after waxing. They can be calmed with an over-the-counter cortisone cream, but you don't need something else to worry about the night before your wedding.

Lightening hair with a peroxide-based cream bleach can be inexpensive and a painless way to deal with light hair growth on legs and upper lip.

Keep in mind that if the hair is very dark, it will lighten to an unattractive dark yellow that is more obvious than natural hair.

Considered the only proven permanent hair removal method, electrolysis zaps hair follicles with an electrical current to kill the hair root. It works about half the time, so treatment needs to be repeated to clear an area of hair. Not painless, and requiring commitment of time and money, it is usually reserved for facial hair problems. To avoid problems of scarring and infection, work with a licensed, well-recommended electrolysis professional.

Believed by some experts to be the most promising development in hair removal since the razor, lasers offer a long-term, if not permanent, solution to hair removal. It not only zaps off existing hairs, it stunts regrowth of new hair. Doctors report that after two or three sessions up to 80 percent of the patients found that hair did not return for more than four months. It is rather expensive, so it is usually used for critical, sensitive areas, such as around the lips, chin, sideburns, and bikini lines. Prices hover around $400 per treatment, and you usually need at least two sessions for each body part.

There are two different laser systems for hair removal. The YAG laser was the first to be approved by the FDA. It is a gentle laser, that requires that the skin be waxed to open the pores, then massaged with a carbon-based lotion. "When the laser passes over the skin, it heats the carbon trapped in the follicles, damaging the hair-growing apparatus," explained Dr. Lefkovits of New York.

The newer, more powerful Ruby laser does not require pretreatment to destroy the hair and hair-germinating cells. Bear in mind that the Ruby lasers can burn darker skins, and they can be ineffective for very light hair. "Because some people are more sensitive to the laser light than others, it is important that you test in a nonsensitive area to see how your skin reacts to the light. If redness fades within a day or so and there's no loss of pigmentation, then you can proceed to use the laser to remove hair on visible areas of your skin," assured Dr. Lefkovits.

Lasers can infrequently temporarily lighten or darken natural skin tones. This problem resolves itself over time, but it's certainly something that you don't want to have to deal with for your wedding. If you are interested in laser hair removal, investigate it at least six months before the wedding date.

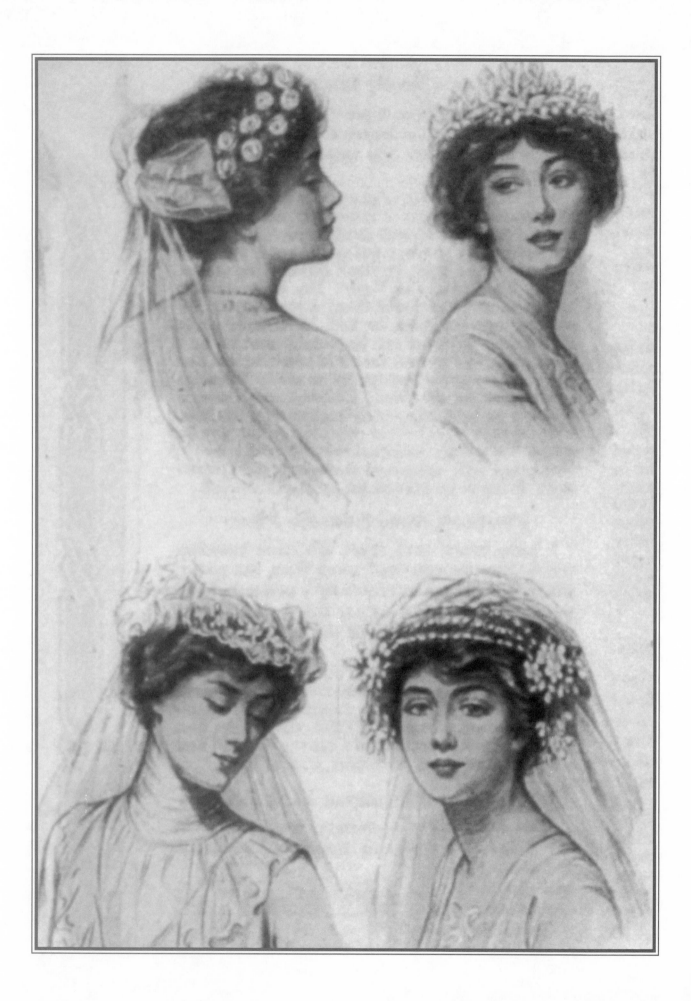

CHAPTER FIVE

The Wedding Ensemble

goals:
....

* **To choose the perfect wedding dress**
* **To select the most flattering headpiece and veil**

From the time you were a child, you probably had an image of yourself in a wedding gown. Perhaps it was a full ball gown covered with lace and pearls. Maybe it was a sleek, bias-cut satin gown that could have been worn by Jean Harlow. When you first start to go shopping for your wedding gown, you may be in for a rude awakening. As you walk into a bridal salon, you may be met by a sea of white dresses that are heavy to try on and rarely ever fit. You'll hear words like Alençon lace, basque waistline, or illusion neckline and not have a clue what they mean.

Shopping for a wedding gown is unlike anything you've ever experienced before, and you need a lot of information and a good strategy to help you find the gown for what should be one of the most glorious days of your life. You will need to balance your childhood fantasy of a wedding gown with the demands of your own wedding style, the strength and weakness of your figure, and the limits of your budget.

Buying the Right Dress

The search for your bridal gown starts by looking through the pages of a bridal magazine. Flag anything that appeals to you, regardless of price, color, or availability. You're trying to find a gown with the magical aura you want.

Marcy Blum, wedding planner and author of *Weddings for Dummies*, suggests keeping in mind the lines of a favorite dress. "It doesn't have to

One of the great joys of a wedding is the opportunity to try on some of the most flattering clothing you will ever encounter. Traditional bridal dresses are created to enhance the female form, not to promote a designer's ego or image. These are user-friendly clothes that don't ask you to starve or spend hours in the gym. Most styles can be counted on to show off creamy shoulders or feminine cleavage as they hide large hips and whittle inches off the waist.

be an elaborate or formal dress. It could even be a simple summer cotton frock, but whatever it is, it is a dress that every time you put it on, you feel good." Think about the individual features. Was it tight through the bodice? Did it have a full skirt? Or was it straight and narrow? Was it sleeveless? Long sleeves? How did the neckline fit against your front and your back? What was it about this dress you enjoyed wearing? Was the fabric soft and comfortable?

Soon you should have a folderful of gowns and feel ready to assault the bridal salon. But before you do so, you need to answer five questions. These are the questions that sales consultants at the bridal salons will be asking. They need this information to help guide you toward the right dress. In most bridal shops, you cannot just pull the dresses off the rack and try them on. Depending on what your answers are, the sales consultant will select the dresses he or she feels meet with your needs. You will notice they don't ask about taste or style as much as the logistics of the wedding.

QUESTION #1: WHAT IS THE DATE OF THE WEDDING?

You do not need to have the exact date, but you do need to know the season. This will determine the fabrics that they will show you, such as a velvet or heavy satin for winter, or a chiffon or organdy for summer. Season is equally important for the sleeve length, whether it is a summery, sleeveless style or a long style suitable for winter. It will also help the sales consultant determine necklines. For example, a Queen Anne neckline with a high collar in the back is very flattering to some figures, but can be far too heavy for warm weather weddings.

QUESTION #2: WHAT TIME OF DAY IS THE WEDDING?

Again, you don't need to know the exact time, but you need to be able to tell the consultant if it will be a morning, afternoon, or evening wedding, because this will influence the formality or informality of the dress. For example, daytime weddings call for a dress with less beading and sparkle than a nighttime wedding dress.

QUESTION #3: HOW MANY PEOPLE ARE ATTENDING THE WEDDING?

You don't need an exact count, but you need an estimate of the size of the guest list. This, too, will determine the formality and informality of the dress at the actual event. For example, a full ball gown style with a long train will look awkward at a small, informal wedding. Similarly, the large wedding with up to two hundred guests is almost by definition formal and calls for a gown that is more than a simple sheath.

QUESTION #4: WHERE IS THE WEDDING GOING TO BE HELD?

This answer is important because it gives the sales consultant not only an insight into the type of dress that's appropriate, but also a clue to your budget. They don't want to keep bringing dresses out that are way below or above the amount that you want to spend for a gown, nor do they want to bring out dresses that are too formal or informal for the occasion. They want the dress to work with the room, not against it. For example, a gold-trimmed historical silhouette with a full train will not work as well in a country club or a waterside setting as it will in a formal ballroom or cathedral.

QUESTION #5: HOW MANY BRIDESMAIDS DO YOU PLAN TO HAVE?

This will give additional clues as to the extent of the wedding. As the saying goes, the bigger the wedding, the bigger the dress.

The Edwardian Bride

The Edwardian era in the first years of the twentieth century was an era that celebrated women. Their clothes, hair styles, makeup, and etiquette honored the image of the beautiful and virtuous woman. For the first time, clothing manufacturers produced ready-made wedding gowns for a growing and socially ambitious middle class. Edwardian gowns were white with long sleeves and often featured high necklines called wedding band collars.

Beneath her floor-length veil, a bride's long hair was dressed in soft, upswept waves. Bridal makeup consisted of rice powder to whiten the skin. The cheeks were equally pale since rouge was considered a sign of a woman with poor morals. Some more adventurous brides darkened their eyelids with the soot from a burnt cork.

Four Pretty Wedding Gowns

Designs by Mrs. Ralston

Drawings by Augusta Reimer

Dress for Shopping Success

When you go shopping for a wedding gown, dress for the occasion. Don't wear your weekend jeans, sweatshirt, and sneakers, because the contrast between this look and any dress you try on will be so extreme that every dress will look either wonderful or too elaborate. You don't have to dress up as though you were going to a cocktail party, but should look as though you're going to lunch at a nice restaurant. Your companions should be equally well groomed, or their perspective will be skewed if the contrast is too great between how they are dressed and how you look in a gown.

Wear a strapless bra or a bustier under your sweater or blouse so you can really evaluate how a gown looks without the intrusion of bra straps. To complete the package, Monica Hickey, of Saks Fifth Avenue, New York, suggests taking a pair of pale pantyhose and an inexpensive pair of white satin shoes in your favorite heel height. "This will give you the best possible foundation to try on dresses. Be sure to wear some makeup and have your hair clean and well styled; it is impossible to judge how a dress really looks on you if your hair is straggly and pulled up with a scrunchie or tucked into a hair clip. You need to look polished and well groomed in order to judge how the gown is going to appear on your wedding day."

It is best to wear clothes that are easy to take on and off. Avoid clothing with a lot of buttons and straps, and shoes that tie. If at all possible, leave your coats in the trunk of your car when going into the bridal salon, because the showrooms tend to get warm and crowded, especially on weekends. To be able to concentrate on looking for the best gown, some brides take along a large shopping bag in which they dump their purses—as well as their companions'—sweaters, scarves, and gloves so there is just one bag to carry, and they don't have to be burdened with additional materials. Wedding gowns are very heavy. Most are at least ten pounds, and you need your hands free to deal with the gowns.

So Many Choices, Only One Wedding

One of the biggest questions that a bride faces when she first starts out to look for a gown is: Who should she take with her? Although choosing a gown is a highly individual decision, it's not something that you want to do alone. Most brides go out at least once with their mothers. If you have a good relationship with her and share the same approach to fashion, your mom can be an invaluable shopping companion. If you want a different or second opinion, take along a close friend. It's especially helpful that she share your body type. If you are 5' 7" and she's 5' 2", you will naturally be attracted to very different styles and not understand the demands of each other's figures.

The worst time to go shopping for a dress is on the weekend. From February through October, the peak season for buying and fitting wedding

quick tip:

The Right Dress at the Right Time

According to Monica Hickey, director of Custom Bridal Designs at Saks, "It is lovely to wear a wedding gown with a bit of sparkle for an evening ceremony: gowns for daytime should be lighter and simpler."

gowns, bridal salons are terribly crowded. Many salons have at least a two- to three-week waiting list for weekend appointments. Unfortunately, for most working women, Saturday and Sunday is the only time that they can go to look for a gown. Some salons have evening hours, and these are less crowded and a good second choice of time. If you can possibly carve out time during the work day, you will find a quiet salon with time and space to try on and evaluate gowns. On Saturdays, because salons have only one or two samples of each gown, you will find yourself waiting for hours to try on a particular dress, while other brides try on and evaluate it. During the week you will have a much easier time of trying on the gowns that you want, when you want.

Shopping for a wedding gown is unlike any other shopping experience you've ever had. The first thing that you will notice is that unless you are a perfect size 8 or 10, none of the gowns fit. Despite the fact that more than half of all brides order gowns in size 14, bridal salons routinely stock sample gowns in 8 or 10. If you are smaller or larger, you will step into the gown, and then the back will be adjusted. If it is too big, it will be clipped into shape with cheerful red and green plastic clothespins. If it is too small, the bridal consultant will calmly pin on elastic straps that can cover up to a five-inch gap, from one side of the dress to the other across your back. Then, if you find a dress that you like, they will order it in your size. This can be somewhat disconcerting because you will never be able to see how the back looks, and since your back is to the wedding guests throughout the entire wedding ceremony, the back is important in a wedding gown.

Another oddity is the fact that bridal sizing is very different than street wear sizing, and bridal gowns are several sizes smaller than traditional clothing. If you routinely wear a size 10, you may easily order a size 12 or 14 wedding gown. This can be disconcerting; just try to think of it as a foreign numbering system rather than a reflection of your own dimensions.

One of the nicest things about shopping for wedding gowns is that you don't have to make up your mind immediately, worried that a gown won't be available when you return. Most gowns that are available at a bridal salon are samples which you try on and are custom-ordered in your size. Rest assured that you can come back and order the gown that you want without fear of losing your options.

Sticker Shock

Then there is the question of price. Designer gowns that are featured prominently in magazines and books can cost from $4,000 to $15,000. Don't despair. With a little investment of time and planning, you can find wedding gowns for every shape, at every budget. Once you determine the style that looks best for you, you can then look for it at the price that you want to spend. In addition to the basic price, most wedding gowns need to have significant alterations to fit your body perfectly, and these alterations can easily tack on an additional $300 to $400 to the price of the gown.

Bridal gowns are usually not custom-made, but they are custom-ordered. Bridal salons will order gowns in sizes that will meet your dimensions, which can then be adjusted individually to be perfectly fitted. Each bridal manufacturer has different sizing and different dimensions: from one manufacturer, the salon might order a size 10; from others they might order a size 6. You need to trust the salon and the people that you work with; they know what they're doing.

Gowns can also be customized with different features. Many salons will give you the option of a dress with or without a train, changing sleeve lengths, trimmings, and necklines. It's a wonderful feature, and allows you to individualize your dress to balance the fantasy of a bridal look with the strengths and weaknesses of your shape.

Sales consultants at bridal salons have to be part wedding planner and part psychologist. They need to try to give you the dress that you want, with the dress that will look best for you, and still work with your

quick tip:

Sample Sales

Once a year, usually in February, many salons and designers hold sample sales of their gowns. Gowns that were originally up to $5,000 are available at 70 percent off, and it is a terrific opportunity to buy a gown for a fraction of the price that you would have had to pay if you bought it on order. However, most of the gowns are samples, meaning they are sizes 8 to 10. And if you are anything more or less than those sizes, and/or are petite, you may be disappointed at a sample sale, finding virtually nothing that you like at all. In addition, because they are samples, they may be quite shop-worn, with lipstick stains, lost beading, and stretching of fabrics. Sample sales are certainly not the best place to start off your wedding search. It is too chaotic, with crowds of people jammed into one giant fitting room. But if you have been looking for a while, have a good idea what type of dress you want, and are average or above-average height in a slim build, you may well find an incredible bargain at such a sale.

existing wedding plans. When they look at the folder of gowns that you like and see that some may not be flattering or appropriate, they may suggest alternatives.

The Six Basic Bridal Silhouettes

Despite a seemingly endless series of white skirts and lace trimming, there are actually six basic wedding gown silhouettes. They flatter different body types and can be modified with a variety of necklines, sleeve lengths, waistlines, fabrics, and trimmings. If you have a fantasy look and the gown in your head is at odds with what seems to be recommended for your wedding style and body type, go ahead and try on anything you wish. Although it is tiring to try on gowns (they can weigh at least ten pounds apiece), get up early, give it your best shot, and try on any gown that appeals to you. By the end of your first visit, it is likely that you will recognize which bridal shapes work best for your silhouette.

Often your fantasy gown will be replaced by a style, one that looks truly beautiful on you. For example, a slim, petite bride had fallen in love with the idea of a boned bodice and full tulle skirt. In the dressing room it didn't look terrible, but there was definitely something missing. The bridal consultant brought in a new style and urged the young bride to "just try it on." When the bride walked out of the dressing room, everyone in the store turned to stare, and her mother started to cry with emotion. The high bateau neck, and the slightly lowered basque waistline added inches to her slight frame. The gently flared skirt with a small sweep made her look delicately regal. It was unlike anything she had pictured in her mind, but the minute she zipped up the button-covered back, she knew that this was the right dress for her wedding.

BRIDAL SILHOUETTE 1: THE BALL GOWN

The ball gown, with a tight bodice, sewn-in waist, and full skirt is sentimental and romantic. In white or ivory satin, it can work beautifully for all body shapes and sizes. With a bouffant tulle or organdy skirt, it is an enchanting look on tall, slim silhouettes. Variations in sleeve style and necklines flatter different body features: for example, a boned bodice is a wonderful look for a small rib cage and high bustline, while a lightly lowered, pointed basque waist chisels off pounds and inches around your middle. As a general rule, your height should be directly proportional to the skirt. That is, the taller you are, the fuller the skirt. The ball gown shape works beautifully for all but the most informal weddings. It can just sweep the floor or be enhanced by a train.

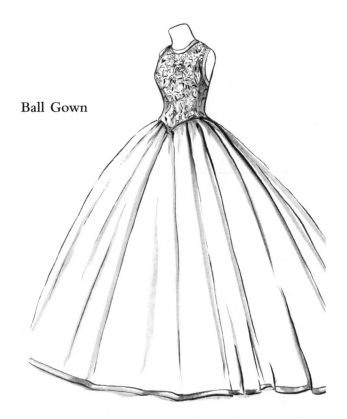

Ball Gown

BRIDAL SILHOUETTE 2: THE PRINCESS/A-LINE GOWN

This body-skimming style, flattering to all shapes, heights, and seasons, was created by the great nineteenth-century designer Charles Worth. The first Princess gown was worn by the Princess of Wales in 1873 in her marriage to Edward, Queen Victoria's eldest son. It is a style that is still popular after more than one hundred years. This style can be worn from informal to ultraformal weddings. The Princess gown is particularly beautiful for petite brides because it creates an unbroken, graceful line that gives an illusion of height.

The Princess can be made in a range of sleeve styles and necklines, each chosen according to a bride's individual taste. For an informal wedding, the Princess gown can just sweep the floor, while an ultraformal ceremony might inspire a gown with a nine-foot-long train. This silhouette can be embellished with lace, embroidery, and crystals (avoid heavy decoration over the bodice if you are busty).

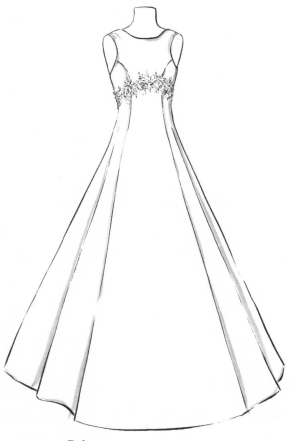

Princess

BRIDAL SILHOUETTE 3: THE EMPIRE GOWN

Inspired by eighteenth-century neoclassicism, the Empire silhouette is another style that works for all heights and weights. This high-waisted design with a skirt that falls directly from the bustline can be worn for all degrees of wedding formality in both cool and warm weather ceremonies. To trim inches off the waist and bust, the Empire waistline should be cut slightly higher in the front and slightly lower in back.

BRIDAL SILHOUETTE 4: THE SHEATH

A body-hugging silhouette with no definite waistline on a slim-line skirt, this narrow, sexy style can be challenging to wear. It is flattering for three somewhat different body shapes. Brides with a slim, well-proportioned body will look beautiful in this body-contouring style. If you have slim hips and waist and a full bosom, you may have found that the full skirted wedding dresses seem to add unwanted pounds and inches. By contrast, the sheath style will create an enviably slim, shapely, hourglass silhouette. Slim, petite brides will be equally flattered by a dress that doesn't seem to overpower them. Intensely feminine, the sheath gown is a favorite choice for small or second weddings. Even embellished with lace or beading, it is not considered enough of a gown for ultraformal ceremonies. A detachable train, however, can be added to enhance formality for a church wedding.

Empire

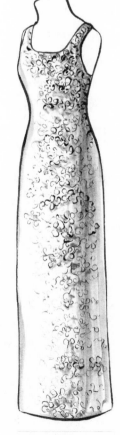

Sheath

BRIDAL SILHOUETTE 5:
THE SLIP DRESS

Immortalized by Carolyn Bessette in her marriage to John Kennedy, Jr., this is an elegant, spare style that needs—no, demands—a tall, slim, well-toned body. The slip dress reveals a great deal of skin, so be certain that the skin on your arms, chest, and back are flawless if you choose this style. Sexy yet elegant, this is the perfect gown for a semi- or informal warm weather wedding.

BRIDAL SILHOUETTE 6:
HISTORICAL GOWNS

Elaborate and dramatic, these gowns feature vintage details, including medieval lacings, high Victorian collars, and antebellum ruffles. They are usually heavily embellished gowns, often decorated with gold trim or constructed of rich brocade. The ornate style and heavy fabrics are best worn by tall, slim brides at formal and ultraformal cool weather weddings.

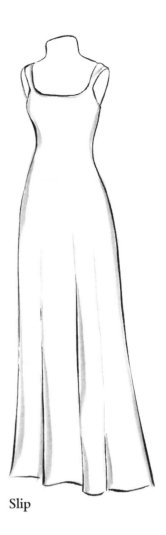

Slip

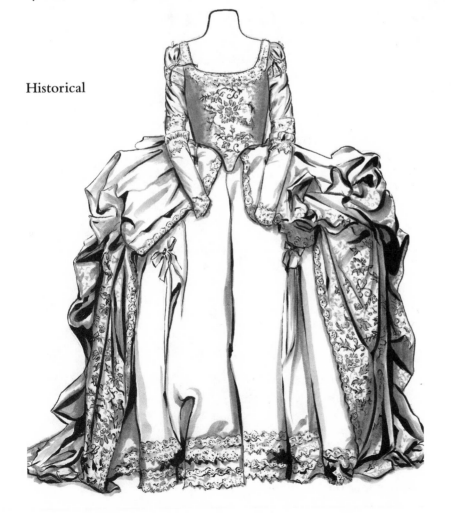

Historical

Bridal Features and Details

The basic silhouette sets the tone and style of the wedding, but it will be the individual details of the neckline, sleeve, and train that create personal style.

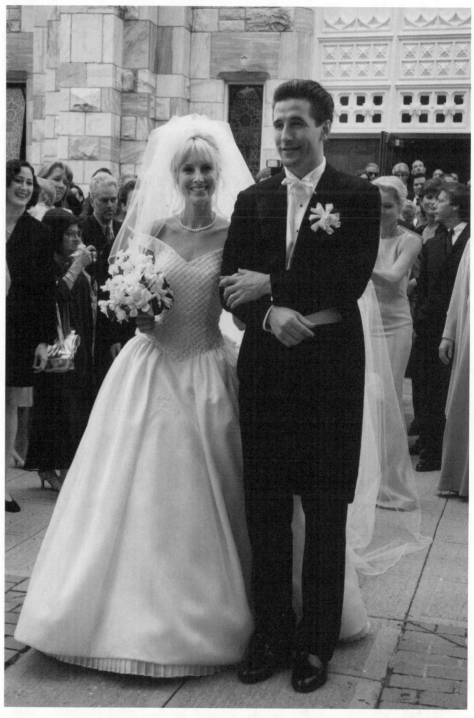

When Chyna Phillips married William Baldwin in 1995, she wore a classic off-the-shoulder gown from Vera Wong. The gown's simple lines were enhanced with beading on the bodice and a long, flowing train.

NECKLINES

The critical focus of a gown, a neckline draws attention to your face and hair. They can change the formality of a gown, as they enhance shoulder, bust lines, and help define a waistline.

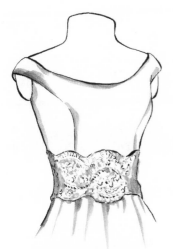

Off-the-shoulder

Off-the-shoulder Neckline:

This is currently one of the most popular styles. It is elegant and flattering to all but the largest bosoms. To maintain the line, the bodice may need to be boned for support. This style is perfect for women with beautiful shoulders and smooth, clear skin. If you tend to become red and splotchy when warm and excited, look for another neckline.

Jewel Neckline:

The jewel neckline works beautifully for informal to ultraformal weddings. So named because it was originally designed as a background for a necklace, the high, round line is popular in cool weather ceremonies.

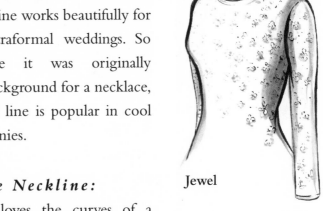

Jewel

Queen Anne Neckline:

This neckline loves the curves of a woman's body. Sculpted to outline bareness at the collarbone and upper chest, it is particularly flattering for full-figured silhouettes. Because of its high collar at the back, it is not the best choice for warm weather ceremonies. Depending on the style of the dress, it can be worn at informal to ultraformal weddings.

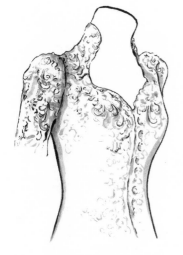

Queen Anne

*Every Bride Is
Beautiful*

Illusion Neckline:

With the scoop of a jewel neck and a sheer, almost invisible bodice, this is an elegant and formal feature. It is usually part of an elaborate gown for an evening ceremony.

Bateau:

A shallow curve across the collar line, bateau was a popular neckline in the 1950s and adds a wonderful retro flavor to a contemporary wedding gown. Good for small frames and narrow shoulders, it can be embellished with beading to create curves.

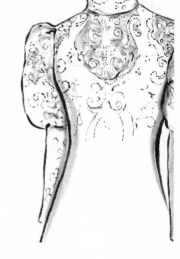

Bateau

Wedding Band Neckline:

This neckline was first popular in the 1890s. This high, fitted collar is an elegant historical style that looks wonderful on tall, thin frames and small bustlines. Because it tends to shorten height, it is not a good choice for petites. The wedding band is usually worn in combination with long, Edwardian sleeves in a sheath or Princess line for a cool weather wedding.

Scoop Neckline:

The scoop neckline is a gentle shape that frames the face with an aura of innocence. The lower curved line is an excellent choice for the bride with a beautiful neck and shoulders. It looks wonderful for average to ample bust lines, but less right for bony or small chests. It can blend with all degrees of both formality and season. The scoop can be worn with virtually all bridal styles, with the exception of a slip dress.

Illusion

Wedding Band

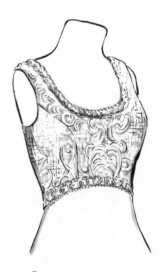

Scoop

V neck:

The V neck angles the fabric to a point, creating a line that flatters a large bosom and slims a too-thick waistline. A plunging V neckline that exposes skin is called "décolletage." Unabashedly sexy, the deep V neck seems to magically slim rounded cheeks.

Sweetheart Neckline:

This neckline, recognized for its ability to chisel pounds and inches from busts and waist, is a gentle, innocent shape that opens up the neck and face. This traditional style was worn by Princess Elizabeth at her marriage to Prince Philip in 1947. Originally introduced in the 1930s, this low neckline is cut to resemble the rounded domes of a heart. It can be adapted to any wedding silhouette except the slip dress, and any season or degree of wedding formality.

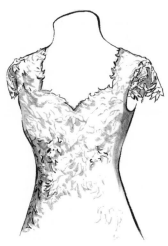

Sweetheart

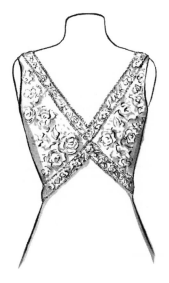

V neck

SLEEVE STYLES

Sleeves provide interest to the bodice and balance the skirt of the gown. Unlike necklines, which can usually be worn in many seasons, sleeve lengths are closely tied to the weather at the time of the wedding.

Sleeveless:

This style works beautifully for slim, well-toned bodies and warm weather weddings. If your shoulders are sloping, albeit your arms are slim, it would be best to look for another style.

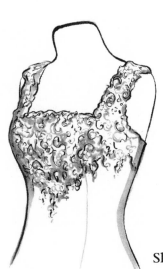

Sleeveless

Every Bride Is
Beautiful

Short Sleeves:

A wonderful summer look for all shapes and sizes, short sleeves can provide an elegant look for informal to ultraformal weddings. They can work well for all body types and are a wonderful compromise for a warm weather bride who feels her upper arms are not her best feature.

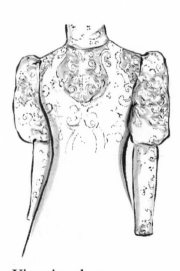

Short sleeves

Long, Fitted Sleeves:

These are an equally wonderful look for winter wedding gowns and hide a multitude of problems. Long and narrow, they usually have a snap or row of buttons at the wrist. Sometimes the long sleeve is finished with the wedding point, a V-shaped extension that comes to a point covering the top of the bride's hand.

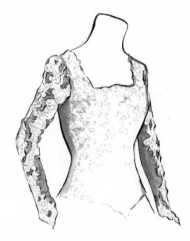

Long sleeves

Juliet Sleeves:

Named for the Shakespearian heroine, the Juliet sleeve is a long, fitted style with a puff at the shoulder. They work best for average and taller heights, and can somewhat overpower a petite frame.

Puffed Sleeves:

These bring a youthful look to petites and add curves to a small bustline. Dainty and charming, they should be avoided if your arms are heavy or if you have a generous bust.

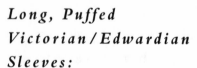

Juliet

Long, Puffed Victorian/Edwardian Sleeves:

These sleeves add a wonderful historical detail for tall, slim, or small-busted shapes. A dramatic sleeve, it is wider and rounder at the shoulder, tapering to a slim fit on the lower arm. Popular for all but informal weddings, it blends beautifully with the wedding band collar, a slim skirt, and a graceful train.

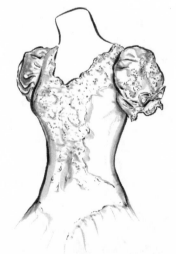

Short, puffed sleeves

Victorian sleeves

THE BRIDAL TRAIN

The sweep of the gown as you walk down the aisle is the detail that makes the bridal gown unique from any other dress you will ever wear. Originated during the Middle Ages, train length indicated rank at court. The longer the train, the greater was your stature with the King and Queen. There are four basic train lengths:

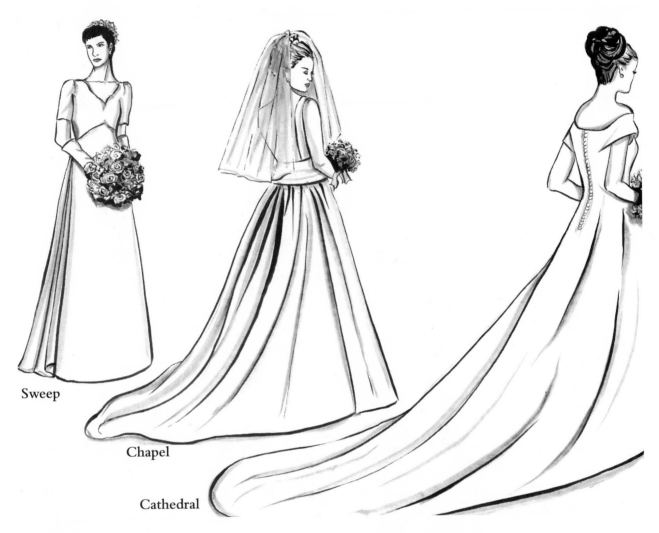

Sweep

Chapel

Cathedral

The Sweep:

Also known as the brush length, the sweep is a modest train that just touches the floor. It is usually worn for semiformal and informal weddings. It looks well with all body shapes and won't overpower a small frame.

Chapel-Length:

This train extends four feet from the waist and flows about one to two feet behind the bride. It works beautifully for semiformal to formal weddings and is the longest style that can be worn by a petite woman.

Every Bride Is Beautiful

Cathedral Trains:

This train, which extends two and a half yards of fabric from the waist, is suitable for formal and ultraformal weddings. Good for average height and frames, it may overpower petite silhouettes.

Royal and Extended Trains:

This is the grandest train of all, sweeping at least nine yards of fabric along the floor. This is the train for the ultraformal wedding, held in a large church or cathedral. As a general rule, wedding consultants feel a big room deserves a "big dress." Lady Diana Spencer wore a twenty-five-foot-long extended train at her wedding at St. Paul's Cathedral.

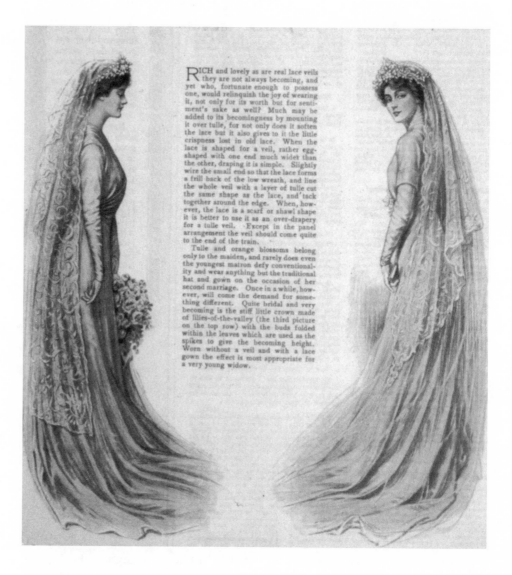

BRIDAL FABRICS

The luminous lustre and drape of a satin silk have made it a favorite bridal fabric for centuries. It is heavy enough to create a full skirt and train, yet light enough to mold to a body's contours. Wrinkle-resistant, it looks as fresh and beautiful at the end of the wedding, when the bride throws her bouquet, as she did when she first walked down the aisle. Different weights and different weaves of silk produce fabrics with unique characteristics that work best with different seasons, degrees of formality, and body types.

Silk Crepe:

Crepe has a dull finish that drapes softly around the body. It works well for short and stocky silhouettes, and it is often used for informal or semiformal warm weather weddings.

Silk Taffeta:

Taffeta has a shiny, stiff finish that flatters tall, thin silhouettes. Traditionally winter weight, it has a lovely rustle as the bride walks down the aisle.

Silk Damask Woven with Floral Patterns:

This was the silk that Marco Polo brought back from the Orient. It has a grandeur that looks beautiful in formal gowns for winter weddings. Best for taller, skinnier silhouettes.

Duchesse Satin:

A blend of silk and rayon, duchesse satin is lighter in weight than satin silk, making it an excellent choice for summer weddings. Arguably the most popular fabric for wedding dresses, it flatters all body weights and heights.

Silk Chiffon:

Described by Coco Chanel as a fluttering breeze, silk chiffon is an enchanting, slimming fabric for spring and summer ceremonies. Designed in simple straight lines, it is a beautiful choice for slim and average silhouettes. Well cut with additional layers of chiffon, it is elegant on heavier frames.

Every Bride Is Beautiful

Peau de Soie:

Translating to "skin of silk," this heavier fabric has a fine, ribbed texture and dull finish. It is an excellent look for slim, winter/autumn brides.

Tulle:

A fabric meshlike weave, tulle is used in layers to create full, graceful skirts, that is an ethereal contrast with a tight satin bodice. Best for tall, slim brides.

Silk Velvet:

Created in Italy at the start of the Renaissance, this fabric adds a lustrous, regal grandeur to winter wedding gowns. Because of its texture and shine, velvet looks best on slim, lean silhouettes.

A DIFFERENT SHADE OF PALE

Bridal fabrics are found in many shades of white. It is important to choose the one that is most flattering to your skin tones. As a general rule, brides with dark eyes and dark hair look best with cool white shades, while blonds with lighter eyes are flattered by creamier off-white tones.

The Perfect Finish: The Bridal Veil

The defining bridal element, the bridal veil is believed to have originated in ancient Greece. Symbolizing purity and virginity, the veil itself can be embellished with pearls, crystals, and the edges trimmed with ribbon or lace. A puff at the back of the veil is a wonderful addition for petite silhouettes, because it adds height. A simple dress can take an elaborate or plain veil, while an elaborate gown should be combined with a simple veil to avoid bridal overload. According to bridal etiquette, it is not appropriate for a bride to wear a veil at a second wedding. There are eight basic styles of veils.

1. The Birdcage or Madonna:

This veil falls just below the chin and is worn at informal weddings.

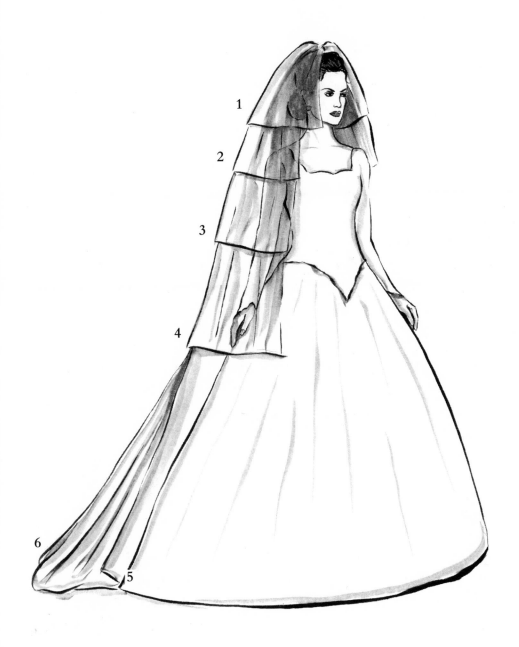

2. Flyaway:

This veil has multiple layers that just touch the shoulder and are best combined with informal ankle-length gowns.

3. Elbow length:

This veil gives a delicate look for informal and semiformal weddings. It is a particularly flattering length for petite brides.

4. Fingertip-length:

This is one of the most popular styles of veil; it is flattering to all heights and appropriate to all but the most ultraformal gowns.

5. Chapel-length:

This veil is seven feet long and works with a dress that is floor-length or with a sweep train. It is worn at semiformal and informal weddings.

6. Cathedral:

This veil is ten feet long and is worn with cathedral-length trains. It is reserved for formal and ultraformal weddings.

7. Blusher:

This veil shades the face as the bride walks down the aisle. Worn in conjunction with other veils, it is lifted up as the ceremony begins.

Mantilla:

The mantilla is a large circular veil made of lace or lace trimmed tulle. This Spanish-inspired veil creates a small neat head and offers a profile-softening silhouette. Formal and regal, is it frequently a family heirloom handed down from generation to generation.

The Headpiece

The ornament which positions the veil on the head, the headpiece is drenched in tradition. Each of the seven most popular, distinct styles comes with its own individual history of myth and ceremony.

Cloth-covered Headband:

Either plain or embellished with decoration, the cloth-covered headband is excellent for medium-to-long hair. It is a wonderful, fresh, youthful look that was probably inspired by the headband worn by Alice in her journey through wonderland. (In England, it is still called an Alice band.) It works beautifully for all seasons and all but the most formal weddings.

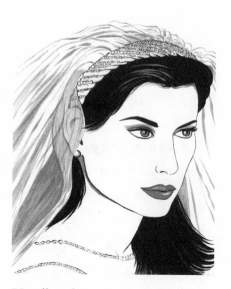

Headband

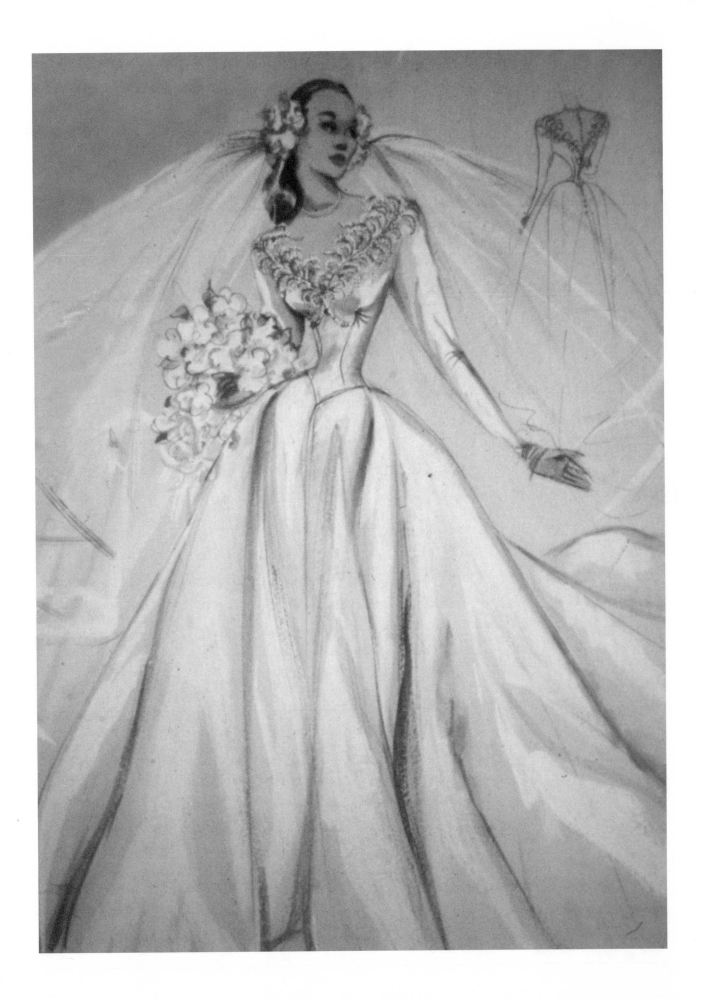

Garland of Flowers:

The garland has been a symbol of bridal virtue since the time of the Druids. Surrounded by a full, layered veil, the garland is a wonderful look for short hair. When tilted low over your forehead, it draws flattering attention to your eyes, making them seem enormous.

Garland

Tiara:

A small delicate crown of pearl and/or crystals, the tiara is the perfect headpiece for all but informal weddings. It works beautifully with Princess line dresses, especially those with higher necklines, continuing the upward line that pulls every eye to the bride's face.

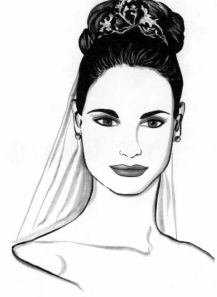

Tiara

Full or Half Circlet:

Made of silk flowers, pearls, and/or crystals, the circlet is a wonderful finish to a gown with a basque waist and scoop neckline. Flattering for medium and long hair up-dos, the circlet is appropriate for all seasons and ceremonies.

Simple Comb:

Decorated with flowers, a bow, crystals, or pearls, the simple comb is currently one of the most popular headpiece styles. By not adding an additional complicated element, a small decorated comb allows the dress to take center stage.

Circlet

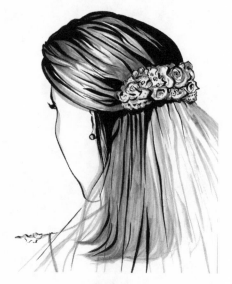

Deborah
Chase

Comb

Picture Hat:

The picture hat is a wonderful outdoor look. Worn without a veil, it is perfect for informal and outdoor weddings.

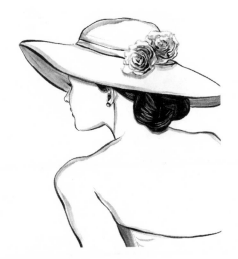

Picture hat

Crown:

A crown reflects the royal origins of the traditional wedding ceremony. The pomp and grandeur of the ceremony, from the processional to the flowing, dramatic trains, are adapted from court ceremonies. A full crown, glittering with pearls and crystals, adds a regal look to formal and ultraformal weddings. It adds a special air of grandeur to low-necked Princess- and empire-style wedding gowns.

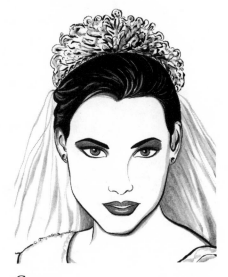

Crown

When you have selected your gown and veil, it is now time to turn attention to bridal hairstyles, makeup, and nail color. As you read through the next chapters, try to visualize yourself in these varied bridal beauty styles. Think about brides you have seen and match the looks you liked to the different hair and cosmetic options that are described in the pages that follow. It is a wonderful opportunity to learn new beauty techniques that you will be able to use for years to come.

YOUR WEDDING

Ask Elizabeth Arden's Bridal Counsellor Service to plan your wedding ...gown, bridesmaids' dresses, coiffures and make-up...and match your flowers with fragrance from Miss Arden's Bride's Bouquet of Floral Perfumes...gardenia, jasmine, lily of the valley, orange blossom or white orchid...Bride's Bouquet of Floral Perfumes, $22.50. Single bottles, $5.50

Elizabeth Arden

CHAPTER SIX

Bridal Makeup

goals:

* ★ **To choose a makeup style**
* ★ **To learn how to execute flawless bridal makeup**

O n your wedding day, you will be the focus of attention. As the star of the day, all eyes will be drinking in every aspect of your appearance. You want
and deserve a makeup that will help you look as beautiful as
you feel. It is equally important that the wedding makeup style
you choose still looks like you. Some brides are tempted to
remake themselves into a more glamorous image—and a good
makeup artist can literally repaint a face with new features and
dimensions. But the most respected wedding consultants, such
as Marcy Blum, caution against such transformations. "You
don't want a look that is different from anything you looked
like before or ever will again," Blum says. "I have seen grooms
go into shock as they watch a woman come down the aisle
that they hardly recognize. This isn't the woman he went out
with, nor the woman he asked to marry. This is a stranger."

To create a memorable and personal bridal beauty style,
you need to understand the special demands of wedding
makeup. Successful bridal makeup needs to look as good in
photographs as it does in person. Your routine day- or nighttime
makeup may look wonderful, but it probably is not the best
choice for wedding photographs. You are going to have the

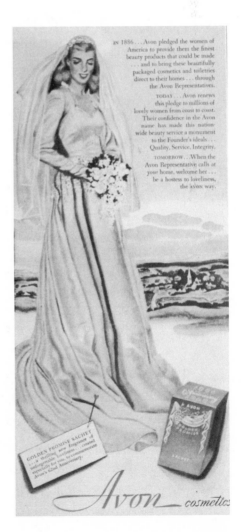

wedding photos in an album for the rest of your life, and you want to look as good in these pictures as you did on the day of the wedding.

There is frequently the dilemma of finding makeup that looks beautiful in photographs, yet is comfortable and easy to wear. If you usually wear very light makeup, the heavier makeup needed for photography may seem unpleasant. You need to balance the needs of photography with your own comfort level. It's your day, and if you are not comfortable, don't let anyone pressure you into using products that you do not want.

Making Up the Bride

Whatever style of makeup you choose, it must last through hours of ceremony and celebration. You will put on wedding makeup several hours before you walk down the aisle and it needs to stay fresh and beautiful for the next twelve hours. As any woman knows, most products tend to wear off within three to four hours. Wedding makeup calls for long-lasting products applied with skill and accuracy. You won't be able to to freshen it during the day, because adding more products will create a messy and blotchy appearance. Unless you are planning to stop dancing and get your face completely redone, the wedding makeup should be created to stay beautiful with a light retouch of lipstick and powder.

To achieve the look you want, you will need to assemble the right tools and products and learn new bridal makeup techniques. As you select the best items for your skin and makeup needs, label them and set them aside in a wicker basket. This will ensure that you will have what you need when you need it.

CLEANSING THE WEDDING-DAY FACE

As you wash your face before the wedding, you are preparing the skin to look beautiful for the next twelve hours. You need thorough yet gentle cleansing that leaves the skin fresh and smooth. The best cleanser for this purpose is a creamy liquid that rinses off with water. Try different formulations before the wedding to select the product that leaves your skin refreshed but not irritated. To assess the effect on your skin, check every two hours and analyze the results. Does your skin feel tight? Does makeup become oily within an hour? Do you feel any itching or eye irritation? Does makeup go on smoothly? When you find a cleanser that leaves the skin comfortable and is compatible with your makeup, buy a fresh bottle of the cleanser, label it, and put it in your wedding-day beauty basket.

THE UNDER BASE

If you have dry skin, you need a moisturizer. If you have oily skin, you need an oil-absorption lotion below your foundation. The moisturizer is not so much to keep the skin moist during the day, but to allow you to apply the makeup smoothly. The oil-absorption factor is to absorb at least some of the oil that you may produce so that your makeup will not just slide off your face within an hour or two. Use either one of these products on a clean face. Apply a small amount and let it absorb into the skin. Wait five minutes before continuing to the next step.

FOUNDATION

A good foundation is the start of any bridal makeup, covering irregularities and smoothing skin color. Matte makeup, which is good for skin that tends to be oily, looks flat without shine. Light-reflective foundation is good for skin that tends to be dry, because it creates a glowing, unlined skin tone. If you have normal or combination skin, you should try both and see which gives you the most luminous and long-lasting glow. There are also new foundations that are formulated to be long-lasting; not only will they stay on through the ceremony and dancing, but they promise not to transfer to your dress or to your groom's collar.

When choosing a foundation, match the color to the skin at the side of your chin. If you are getting married in the summer, or tend to flush when you get excited, look for a foundation that is slightly lighter than your skin tone. If you become flushed during the wedding, a too dark foundation will tend to look hot and sweaty in photographs, a lighter foundation will even out the skin tones. Bridal makeup experts, such as Laura Geller, suggest that if you are in doubt about the color, choose a lighter shade in most cases.

To Tan or Not to Tan

It's unequivocally true that a tan makes you look more healthy and rested. It covers up imperfections in the skin and seems to slim the contour of the face. But for a bride, a tan is not the most flattering tone. In photographs, tans tend to make the skin look muddy and sweaty. It can actually create unattractive shadows, and the skin can look leathery and toughened. A fake tan is no better; it makes the skin look greasy in photographs. Unless you are a person who people never see without a tan, a tan is not recommended for the wedding day. If a tan is your signature look, you are probably going to be interested in an informal or semiformal outdoor wedding, where the sunlight, sand, and a casual gown will work spectacularly together.

You have foundation choices of liquid, cream compact, or stick formulation. Liquids that provide a natural coverage are formulated for all skin types. They supply the least coverage and should be used on skin that is in good condition and without significant problems to cover. They work well for people who don't like wearing makeup and are not used to the sensation on their skin. The one type of foundation that you will probably have less success with is oil-free shake lotions. They don't provide that much coverage, and they will not give you the smooth, luminous glow that you want for both the photographs and the actual ceremony.

Cream foundations are often formulated for drier skins, and they provide a somewhat heavier coverage. They are good for all but oily skin. Cream compacts provide heavier coverage and are always applied with a moist sponge. Although they have a heavier—almost oily—consistency, they can actually be drying to fine, thin skins. They provide excellent coverage if you have blemishes, discolorations, or broken blood vessels in your skin.

The heaviest coverage is available with stick foundations, which are actually a combination of a cream and a concealer. These products can hide almost anything in photographs, including scars and birthmarks, and they are a good product to have on hand in case you have an unexpected eruption of blemishes.

Whatever type you use, the best way to apply foundation is with a latex sponge wedge, because the points can get into the corners of the eye and even off small areas on the contours of the chin better than a rounded sponge.

FACE POWDER

Powder is an essential component of the bridal makeup. Even if you never wear powder, it is important to fix the foundation and have it last through the wedding activities. Happily, powder takes away shine without creating a thick, over-made-up look, and can be reapplied during the day without causing a buildup. Loose powder is a favorite of most makeup artists: it is applied with a brush, and then the excess is dusted off. There are two schools of thought about powder. Some use an almost translucent powder, and that's good if your skin is pale. Others swear by a yellow, sheer powder that is good for all skin tones. It cools off ruddy skin and blends beautifully with pale or olive complexions.

CLOSE-UP:
The Jazz Age Bride

The sea changes in the social fiber that began during World War I forever altered the status of women. First to go was elaborate, time-consuming long hair, which was replaced by short, easy-care cropped styles. Dresses grew progressively shorter and corsets were abandoned. In the early 1920s Chanel introduced the first knee-length wedding dress, accompanied by a full veil that puddled luxuriously on the floor. It combined the modern silhouette with traditional bridal fabrics and it became the most popular wedding gown style of the decade.

The Jazz Age bride enjoyed using makeup. While skin was still pale and powdered, she would blend rouge on her cheeks and tint her mouth with lipstick. Eyebrows were plucked to a pencil-thin line and darkened with a soft black pencil.

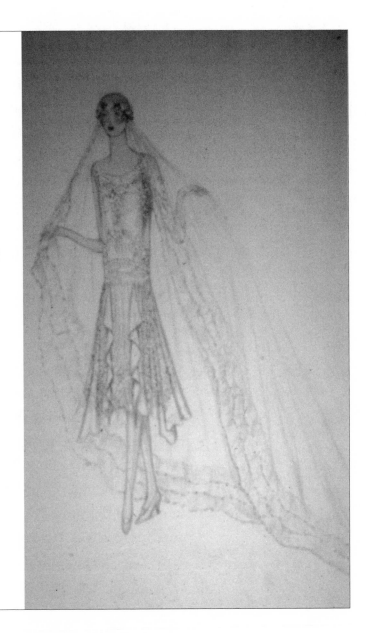

CONCEALERS

Concealers hide what foundation doesn't, including broken blood vessels, under-eye circles, and signs of breakouts. Concealers are available in a range of shades and formulations. Tube concealers provide light coverage, while sticks have a thicker consistency and hide problems more thoroughly. You need to balance the coverage of the concealer with the needs of your skin type. Some of the heavier concealers can be drying for fine, thin skin, while lighter products tend to slide off oily skins. Keep trying different products until you find the right formulation for your needs. For best results, choose a concealer that is slightly lighter than your foundation. Always buy your foundation first and then choose your concealer.

BLUSH

Adding both definition and a natural glow, blush for a wedding needs to be especially subtle. It should be flattering, feminine, and not too dark, because the bridal look is luminous and somewhat pale. It is also important to remember that blush doubles in intensity in color photographs. To avoid looking like a painted doll, use a light hand with your blush brush. Blush should be applied in the natural areas of color high on the cheek. Cream blush can be a problem for oily skin and large pores, and may look too intense in photographs. Powder blush works well for all skin types, and it is easy to control intensity, placement, and reapplication. Gels create a long-lasting, waterproof natural glow but cannot be reapplied over powder to freshen the makeup during the day.

LIPSTICK

Providing color and definition, this is the most obvious part of the bridal makeup. Brown lipsticks should be avoided, even if it's your favorite day-time color. Brown photographs badly, giving you a thin, dark mouth with corners that seem to droop. According to noted makeup artist Laura Geller, reds can be a problem too, because the contrast of the red mouth is too strong with the white gown, and you can look like a pair of lips in a white dress. "If red lipstick is your signature look, you can wear a matte rather than shiny formulation to lessen the contrast," she said confidently.

The most attractive and commonly used lip colors are roses and pinky corals. You can use either a matte or shiny texture, depending on your preference. The lipstick is not only the most obvious cosmetic you are going to use, it's the one that gets the greatest wear and tear. You want to put on a lip color that is going to last as long as possible so it doesn't smear, disappear, or transfer itself to your groom or your dress.

Start with a lip base as a foundation for your lip color. On top of that, use a lip liner, not only to outline the shape, but to completely color in the entire mouth. This gives you a base of color on which you can put your creamier rose or coral. On top of your lip color, if you want to emphasize a slightly pouty look, brush a small amount of lip gloss in the center. In this method you will never completely lose all your lip color, and it is easy to retouch with your basic rose color.

quick tip:

Dark Circles

If you have very dark circles under your eyes, try brushing on a small amount of red-orange lipstick instead of using a skin tone concealer. As outrageous as this sounds, the red cancels out the bluish gray color under the eye far better than a light tone concealer. Brush it on until it's just a pinkish color on your skin and then cover that with your normal foundation. It gives you a naturally fresh, youthful, healthy look.

It's not a good idea to mix different colors to create the perfect lip shade, because you're going to need to reapply lip color during the wedding day. It's very cumbersome to carry several lipsticks and try to remix them in the original color. You're much better off finding a rose or coral long-lasting color that you like and stay with it the whole day. Your bridesmaid or maid of honor should carry your lipstick for you in her glove or purse and then give it to you to reapply, watching out to see that your makeup is fresh. Alternately, some florists can design a little receptacle in the bouquet itself to hide the lipstick, and you can pull it out and adjust your lip color.

EYE MAKEUP FOUNDATION

For the bridal makeup you want to create a full, round, beautiful eye that reflects your joy. To do so, you should start off with an eye makeup foundation. This will prevent the eye makeup from disappearing too quickly. The moisture around the eye, either oil or water, tends to wear out eye makeup quickly or have it run down the corners of the eye. By using an eye foundation, it will stay in place.

THE EYELINER

Eyeliner defines the eyes, making them rounder and well shaped. Liquid liner is long-lasting and doesn't smudge. It creates an elegant, dramatic look. If you have difficulty applying a smooth, liquid line, lay down a line of connecting dots. Pencil lines provide soft focus around the eye, but may smudge on oily skins. New, long-lasting formulations work well in hot weather to avoid smearing.

The eyeliner shade you choose depends as much on your own personal bridal style as on your coloring. A romantic look works beautifully with a navy pencil, while a contemporary bride can use a black liquid liner for a more dramatic look.

MASCARA

Everyone in the bridal party should wear waterproof mascara, because people tend to tear up from happiness and/or stress. Black mascara is good for everyone, while brown is a wonderful choice for a natural, sporty look. To keep the mascara from flaking off onto the rest of the face, finish your colored mascara with a coat of colorless mascara. It fixes the first coat, to make your eyes look enormous, framed with a memorable fringe.

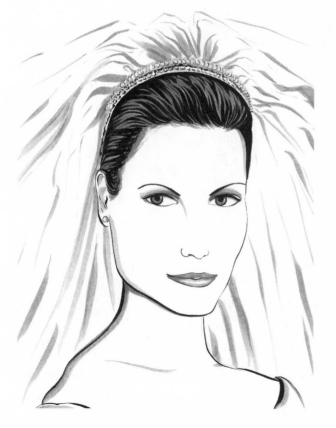

Trying Out Different Looks

The wedding look itself is different from street wear or even party wear. The two most important facts are (1) you must look luminous and (2) the makeup has to be long-lasting. Before the wedding, give yourself time to try out different styles and products. Go to the cosmetic counters, describe your gown and the colors you want to wear, and then ask the makeup consultant to demonstrate their products for you. Studies have shown that brides spend more on cosmetics than at any other time in their lives. In order not to waste your time or money, it's helpful to get an idea of the different bridal looks and how they would apply to your own wedding style.

THE ROMANTIC BRIDE

The romantic bride, decorated with ruffles and lace, is an innocent, gentle look with a youthful glow. The foundation is soft, even, and fairly sheer. You want to make sure that your lipstick is dusty pink rather than brownish pink and that your lipstick and your blush has pink rather than brown or coral undertones. A very dark blue pencil lining both the upper and lower eyelids is an enchanting finish.

1. Apply eye makeup base primer to eyelids and balm to lips.
2. Apply dark blue liner on lower lids and upper lids.
3. Smudge edges for a softer look. Brush taupe shadow on lids up to eye crease and pale peach on the brow bone.
4. Apply foundation with pointed latex sponge.
5. If there are blemishes to cover, use concealer and then top with a bit more foundation.
6. Curl eyelashes.
7. Apply black mascara covered by clear mascara.
8. Apply cream concealer under the eyes, if needed.
9. Smooth on lip foundation.
10. Outline lips in nude and color in the entire surface.
11. Apply coral pink lipstick to the entire surface.
12. Use a touch of gloss in the center.
13. Define eyebrows with brow gel and brush smoothly.
14. Dust a pale peach rose blush on the top of the cheeks.
15. Dust entire face with powder and brush off excess.

THE TRADITIONAL BRIDE

The traditional bride has an almost ethereal, luminous look with a pale yet radiant foundation. With most hair colors, a deep violet eyeliner and a touch of lavender in the shadow is the perfect echo of the flowers and formality of the traditional gown. Lip colors should stay in the rose shades.

1. Apply concealer under the eyes and shadow foundation on the lid and under brow area.
2. Brush in concealer under lash line.
3. Apply lip balm or lip foundation to soften lips, but no other lip color at this time.
4. Apply nude pink shadow on lid and lilac shadow in the crease.

5. Apply small amounts of mauve eye shadow to the outer corner and smudge the edges.

6. Use a violet eyeliner pencil under lower lashes; brush gray shadow over violet eyeliner.

7. Use a violet eyeliner pencil on the bottom of the upper lids.

8. Curl the eyelashes, holding for ten seconds.

9. Apply one coat of mascara, allow to dry for a moment or two, and separate lashes with an eyelash comb. Apply mascara to both upper and lower lids. Wait a moment and apply clear mascara on upper and lower lids to add body and shine—but not extra color.

10. Apply dusty rose powder blush to the apples of the cheek.

11. Outline lips with a mauve or copper pencil.

12. Apply lipliner all over the lips, so that it doesn't create a harsh outer line when the rest of the lip color wears off.

13. Apply a long-lasting, dusty pink lipstick to the entire lips.

14. Top with small area of lip gloss in the center.

15. Groom brows with gel.

16. Brush on pale powder over entire face with full brush and dust off excess.

THE EUROPEAN BRIDE

The European look is slightly more dramatic. The eyes are darker, with more shadow and more distinct eyeliner. The foundation is flawless, while the lipstick tends to be darker. Wedding gowns are often very dramatic with historical notes and gold or silver trim that complement stronger, darker makeup.

1. Apply eye shadow primer to lids.

2. Pencil on smoky gray eyeliner on upper and lower lids, extending lightly.

3. Apply dark shadow on lids and dark gray shadow in the crease and outer edge of the eyes.

4. Use shell pale pink highlighter on the brow bone.

5. Apply a cream foundation for flawless finish.

6. Curl eyelashes and coat with separate coats of black mascara, drying and separating between each application.

7. Use cream concealer under the eyes or where needed.

8. Over your lip base, pencil in the lips in nude pencil.

9. Apply pale, tawny lipstick.

10. Redraw lips with liner.
11. Dot a dab of lip gloss on the center of the lower lip.
12. Apply tawny blush to cheeks.
13. Dust face with powder and brush off excess.
14. Groom brows with gel and brush in shape.

THE CALIFORNIA BRIDE

The California bridal look is a natural, light look. This is the sun-drenched outdoor wedding, and you don't want heavy makeup. You need just enough so that photographs look good, but you want the natural health of your skin to shine through. This will be makeup that uses the lightest liquid foundation, perhaps even a tinted moisturizer—if the skin is clear and smooth. The lipstick should be a dusty rose with a touch of brown, and the blush is a light tan rather than pink. Eyes should not be heavily shadowed but framed with a soft brown pencil, and eyelashes should be curled and colored with dark brown mascara to create a flattering fringe.

1. Apply eye makeup base primer to lids and balm to lips.
2. Line eyes with taupe pencil.
3. Spot on foundation where needed.
4. If your skin is dry, use a tinted moisturizer.
5. Curl eyelashes and apply one coat of dark brown mascara; top with one coat of clear mascara.
6. Apply a light dusting of yellow tone powder over face.
7. Brush on tawny pink blush in the apples of the cheek.
8. Apply lip foundation.
9. Line lips with tawny peach or dusty pink pencil.
10. Apply tawny peach lipstick.
11. Smooth a large dollop of lip gloss in the center of the mouth.
12. Smooth gel on brows.

THE CONTEMPORARY BRIDE

The contemporary bride is a look of polished yet casual elegance. Wonderful for second or informal weddings, this is the one bridal situation where you can wear a sheer, red lipstick, because there is not that much of a big, white dress to create the huge contrast between the lips and the dress. Beautiful doe eyes (think Audrey Hepburn) are a wonderful look for the contemporary bride. The skin should have a flawless foundation but can use a little more color on the cheeks than that worn by the traditional or romantic bride.

1. Apply an eye makeup base primer to lids and balm to lips.
2. Cover lid with bone shadow up to the brow.
3. Apply taupe eye shadow at crease and outer corners of the eyes.
4. Apply bone highlighter under the brow.
5. Stroke on black eyeliner, under and above the eyes, in two lines that meet slightly in the outside corner.
6. Apply foundation with pointed latex sponge.
7. Use concealer where needed.
8. Dust on a pale rose blush.
9. Brush on a translucent powder to the face. If your skin tends to be dry, apply it just to center of face.
10. Brush on black mascara, using two coats. Dry and separate the lashes between each coat.
11. Line lips with red liner.
12. Apply matte red lipstick.
13. Reapply liner to keep lipstick within the line.
14. Dab on drop of lip gloss in center.

THE ASIAN BRIDE

The Asian bride has smooth, almost poreless skin with yellow skin tones. By tradition, Asian brides like pale skin tones and should use foundation one shade lighter than natural skin tones. It is important to stay away from pinks or oranges and use more subtle corals or dusty rose colorings for her lips and cheeks. Eyes need to be carefully lined with a liquid black or smoky gray eyeliner, and a darker, smoky gray shadow is wonderful on the lid. The best color for the cheeks would be a dusty plum blush.

1. Apply eye makeup base primer to lids and balm to lips.
2. Apply black eyeliner to the upper and lower lids.
3. Blend in dark gray shadow, lightening color toward the brow.
4. Highlight brow bone with ivory shadow.
5. Smooth on foundation with pointed latex sponge.
6. Curl eyelashes.
7. Stroke on two coats of black mascara, drying between each coat.

8. Separate lashes with comb.

9. Outline lips with rose lip pencil.

10. Pencil in rest of lips to create even color base.

11. With brush apply tawny pink lipstick.

12. Apply dab of lip gloss in center of lower lip.

13. Brush yellow tone powder on face and dust off excess.

CLOSE-UP:

The Japanese Bride

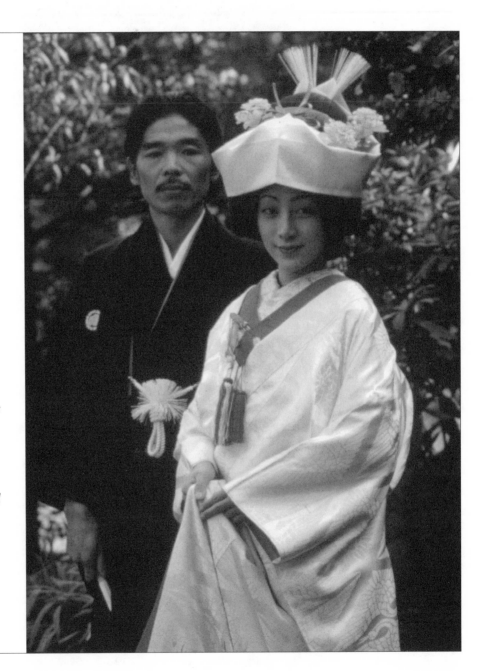

The traditional Japanese bride wears a thick white foundation and has a penciled-in small red mouth. She begins the ceremony in a white silk kimono, changing into a red silk kimono lavishly embroidered with Japanese folk symbols to greet her guests after the ceremony. Her hair is covered by a tall, stylized wig decorated with tortoise shell combs, the turtle being a symbol of long life and many children.

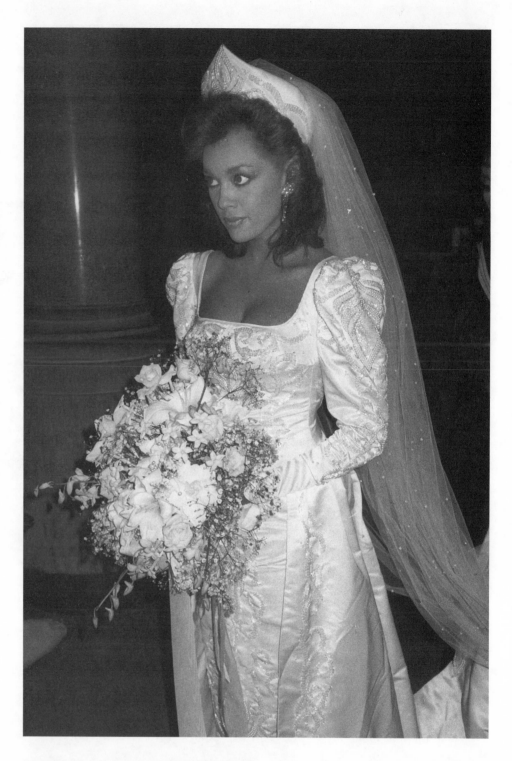

THE AFRICAN-AMERICAN BRIDE

The African-American bride has a vast range of natural skin tones that are mixed pigments of yellow and brown shades. Red tones should be avoided, focusing on the deep plum and berry shades for the lips and cheeks. Blush should be applied with a very light hand. Depending on natural pigments, African-American brides will look best with dark brown or black eyeliner and shades of taupe and brown eye shadows.

1. Apply eye makeup base primer to eyelids and balm to lips.
2. Edge eyes with black eyeliner.
3. Smudge edges and apply plum shadow to lower lids.
4. Brush bone shadow on brow bone.
5. Smooth on foundation that matches the neck.
6. Curl eyelashes.
7. Stroke on black mascara.
8. Separate lashes with comb.
9. Cover lashes with clear mascara.
10. Outline lips with burgundy lip pencil.
11. Pencil in rest of lips to create an even base of color.
12. With a brush, apply burgundy lipstick.
13. Define eyebrows with gel and brush smooth.
14. Dust face with power and brush off excess.

Skillful Bridal Makeup

No matter which makeup techniques you use for this day, it is important that you don't create layer upon layer of contouring with different colors of blushes. This is a professional's work, and unless you have a professional makeup artist with you all the time and take the time out from your wedding to have your makeup redone, you will get splotches of different colors in an unattractive patching. You must pick the colors that you want to use for blush, lipstick, and eye shadow, and then reapply them simply during the day.

If you are going to use black-and-white photography, you'll need to modify each makeup technique slightly. In black-and-white photographs, blush will appear as a contour—so your cheeks will have shadows. In this case you should apply your blush as a contour, below the apples of your cheek.

The Rest of the Wedding Party

Your bridesmaids should wear makeup in the same tone and style as yours, that is, if you have a European look, all the bridesmaids should have a European look. If you're a traditional bride, they should have the traditional, ethereal makeup. The type of foundation can be adjusted to their skin and skin tone, but if you are wearing matte, they should all have matte and if you are wearing a reflective makeup, they should all be reflective. This helps

Bridal Makeup Shopping List

Eye makeup base
Foundation
Concealer
Powder
Eyeliner
Eye shadows
Blush
Brow gel
Mascara
Clear mascara
Lip base
Lipstick
Lipliner
Lip gloss
Latex sponges
Eyeliner pencil sharpener
Eyelash curler
Tweezers
Eyebrow brush
Lash separator
Cotton swabs
Blush brush
Powder brush
Lipstick brush
Eye shadow applicator
Eyeliner sharpener
Eye makeup remover for
    waterproof mascara

create a consistency in photographs, so that everyone looks great. The photographer will adjust the exposure and the lighting to flatter the bride, and if the bridesmaids have different types of foundation, they will look less attractive than they want.

Eye makeup should be customized for eye shape. Deep-set or small eyes should wear lighter shadows on the lids, with darker tones on the outside of the eyes. Prominent eyes need darker shadows on both the upper and lower lids.

There are two schools of thought about lipstick for the bridal party. While all experts agree that the bridesmaids should match the texture (i.e., matte or creamy) the color is a different story. Some feel that each bridesmaid should use the same color as the bride, while others feel the lipstick shade can vary to suit the coloration of each girl. It's a good idea to take the bridesmaids with you to try out makeup in the months before the wedding.

If you and the wedding party are doing your own makeup, there should be plenty of mirrors in the dressing rooms and everyone should have their own supply of products and tools. It's a nice idea to provide a complete wedding makeup kit as a gift to each bridesmaid. They will appreciate your thoughtfulness and it frees you from worrying about whether or not they're going to have the colors and equipment they will need.

Working with a Pro

To polish your makeup application skills, look into lessons with a professional. Most major cosmetic companies offer instruction and free application at their department store counters. Clinique and Macy's offer an annual free bridal clinic while Estee Lauder spas provide makeup lessons and application with the fee applicable to purchase of Estee Lauder products. Such services allow a bride to experiment with a range of makeup styles and products. To evaluate results, carry a disposable camera. It will tell you how well the colors and techniques work for you in photographs.

For a flawless, stress-free makeup, many brides are now hiring a professional makeup artist for private lessons or to apply the makeup on the wedding day. You will need to consult with them months before the wedding to evaluate their style, skill, and approach to wedding makeup. Some of them will do a consultation without charge, but many charge a fee—however, it's worth it to see how well you like the results.

Some artists have one look that they use for their brides. Other artists understand the different bridal styles and will work with you to develop an individual look. You need to see how they work with your features and, more important, the effect of their products and colors on your skin.

If you are having a morning or afternoon wedding, the makeup artist should come to you. The hours before a daytime wedding are far too hectic to accommodate a trip to the salon. With an evening wedding you have the option of visiting a salon (great if they also do hair) or book a home visit. When you use a makeup artist for the entire wedding party, keep in mind that it takes about an hour to do each face. If there are more than two bridesmaids, you will need additional makeup artists to avoid a time crunch.

The mothers of both the bride and groom do not need to wear the same makeup style as the bride and the wedding party. They can wear the colors and styles that are most flattering to their features and age to look as beautiful as possible at the wedding and in the photographs. Getting their faces and hair done with the bride and bridesmaids is a wonderful way to bring generations and families together on this wonderful day.

Insist on

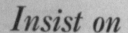

Gainsborough
Genuine HAIR NET

The Net of the Life-Like Lustre

Matchless in Quality
Yet only 10 cents
Everywhere

Gainsborough Double Cap, 15 cents each or 2 for 25 cents.
Gainsborough Double Fringe, 15 cents each or 2 for 25 cents.
Gainsborough White or Gray, 20 cents each.

Ask for this package. For sale by the better stores everywhere.

THE WESTERN COMPANY
402 W. Randolph St.
Chicago

WECO Product

Completes the Hairdress

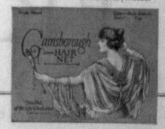

CHAPTER SEVEN

Bridal Hairstyles

goal:
....

★ **To choose the bridal hairstyle that works beautifully with your gown and headpiece as it flatters your face and hair**

We ask a lot of bridal hair styling. In addition to being flattering to your face, it needs to work well in photographs, accommodate your veil and headpiece, and stay beautiful after hours of ceremony and celebration. It's a challenge to arrive at a practical, beautiful bridal style, but with some basic concepts and a few new techniques, it can be achieved by any bride.

Short Versus Long: The Eternal Bridal Hair Debate

As soon as they become engaged, many brides are advised to start growing their hair. There are quite a few bridal experts who believe longer hairstyles are better suited for the bridal look. Others feel that sleek, short hair is a youthful and modern look. If you have a short, charming style that is flattering to your face, it can be worn with a wide variety of dress and headpiece options to create a dazzling bride.

The key, however, is balance. Short hair gives you a small, neat head that works beautifully with contemporary, tailored gowns. Other styles of gowns can pose some problems. An off-the-shoulder or very low-cut wedding gown can create a large, empty space between your ears and your bosom when your hair is short. Gowns that contain historical details, such

The Depression-Era Bride

....

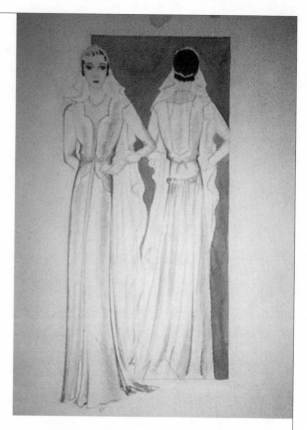

Marriage in the 1930s was a symbol of faith and optimism in a dark, difficult time. Wedding dresses reflected the new austerity. Elaborate, knee-length gowns with pearls, lace, and yards of fabric were replaced by slim, untrimmed, bias-cut floor-length silk dresses. Makeup was frequently the one area that a bride would indulge herself. Now that it was considered socially acceptable to wear cosmetics, many women would not leave their homes without wearing lipstick. Despite its popularity, there were really only two colors—red or a rather atonishing shade of orange—and both were worn for weddings. The bride's short, slightly waved hair would be covered by a broad headband and long veil.

as a high Victorian collar or long, full, medieval sleeves, usually work best with equally romantic, longer hairstyles.

If you have short, layered hair, you may have some difficulty if these layers are designed to give volume and body to the style. Many headpiece styles will flatten the hair unattractively. This is especially a problem if you have full, rather than chiseled, cheeks. A round face, with a round head-piece, on a rounded hairstyle creates too many circles, a look that is bulky rather than beautiful. If this is your regular style, you may want to grow your hair.

Very short hair can be limiting if you are planning to wear a cathedral-length train and veil. The veil will flow toward the back of the head and not be available to frame the face. It can also pose problems for second weddings, where veils are not considered appropriate. Without a veil most headpiece styles perch awkwardly on top of very short hair.

Short hair should be cut and colored (if necessary) about a week to ten days before the ceremony, so that the cut is fresh but not harsh. The headpiece for short hair should not compress or flatten the style. Headbands and heavy crowns tend to distort the lines of short hair as it frames the face. One of the prettiest short-hair looks is a small headpiece such as a bow or flower attached to a comb and attached to the back of the head. This allows the hair to fall freely about the face without being compromised.

If your hair is boyishly short, another beautiful bridal look uses a full wreath of flowers, worn low on the forehead, that covers all but the top of the head. A full veil attached to this wreath supplies the softness and volume that would come from longer hair. This look was worn beautifully by Nadia Comaneci when she wed fellow gymnast Bart Connors in an ultraformal state ceremony in Romania. She wore an off-the-shoulder cathedral-length gown and train, while her wreath of flowers held a cathedral-length veil, creating a soft, regal look that was perfect for the gold-leaf-decorated hall.

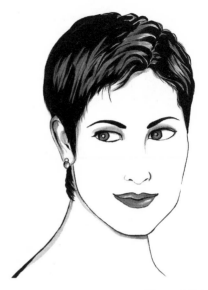

Short Hair

Nadia Comaneci

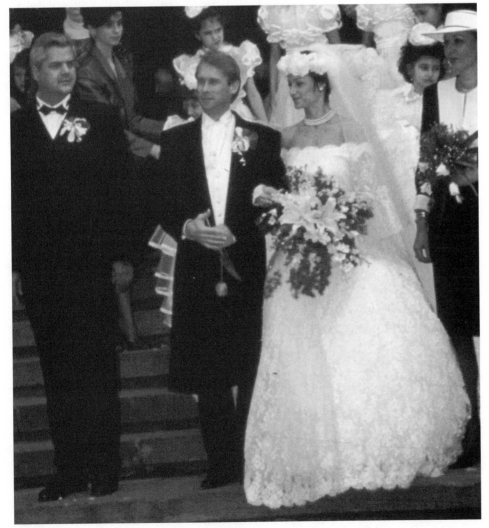

Every Bride Is Beautiful

125

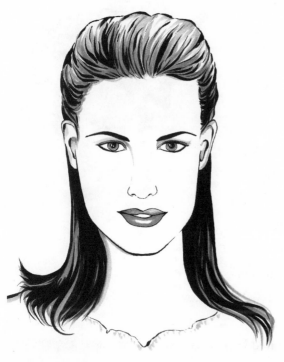

Half and Half

THE BASIC THREE BRIDAL CHOICES

With medium to long hair, there are three standard options: up, half-and-half, and down. Up means the hair is pulled off the face and neck and arranged on the head in a variety of styles, including a high chignon or a graceful back-swept French twist. Half-and-half simply means the top and sides of the hair are pulled up and back in the youthful schoolgirl look that has been a classic bridal style since Victorian times.

When the hair is completely loose and free, it is regarded as "down." This style works best with hair that is medium-length rather than long enough to fall to the shoulders. All three basic styles can be varied with different treatments of front styling and bangs.

THE MANY LOOKS OF MIDLENGTH HAIR

Midlength hair is defined from chin-length to about the bottom of the neck. If you want to wear your hair down, midlength is the perfect style. It is long enough to provide soft volume to frame the face yet short enough to clear the collar and stay fresh and neat. Half-and-half in midlength means the top and crown and sides are pulled back, and the bottom hair is left free—either turned up or under. It is a neat, elegant style that works beautifully with straight hair. Practically every headpiece style works with midlength hair.

If you want to wear your hair up, even if it's barely long enough to make a ponytail, it can still be styled into romantic up-do. The back can be folded into a French twist and the top arranged in barrel curls or a chignon.

LONG HAIR: SO MANY CHOICES, ONLY ONE WEDDING DAY

If you have truly long hair, that is, shoulder-length or longer, you have a range of up-dos and options. In fact, the beautiful styles that are available from French twist to chignon are the reason that many brides do start

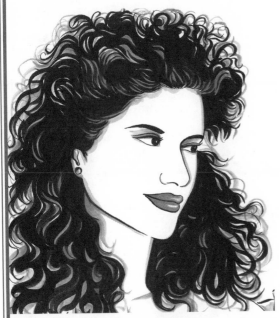

Curly hair:

If you have naturally curly hair, you have an extraordinarily wide range of styling options. If you want to wear it down with loose, free curls, it should be shampooed and conditioned the day before the wedding. Don't brush it out, because that creates unwanted frizz. Towel it dry and scrunch your hair to maintain volume and curl. If you want to smooth out your curls so that you can create a sleek up-do, you need to first set it on hot rollers to regulate line and texture. If your hair has a particularly wiry texture, it can be smoothed and softened after removing the rollers by styling with an electric brush. This will create a softness and hold the line as if you had chemically straightened it. When you wash your hair following the ceremony, it will become curly again.

growing their hair on the day they become engaged. Long hair can be worn half-and-half, with crown pulled back, either flat or full. The ends can hang straight, curl under, or drape into curls. Loose, long hair looks beautiful with a picture hat. To avoid clutter, the dress should be low-neck and/or off-the-shoulder.

Choosing the Bridal Style That's Right for You

The best bridal style depends on weighing four factors: what is flattering to your face; the texture of your hair; the style and fabric of your gown; and the formality or informality of your wedding. If your face tends to be round, you'll probably find it flattering to wear your midlength hair down or half-and-half. The presence of some hair at the side of the cheek will tend to give a slimmer plane to the face, while a full up-do can actually accentuate the roundness. By contrast, a long, thin face needs bangs or fullness at the crown to soften the lines at the forehead.

Certain situations seem to demand an up-do. They are an ideal choice for outdoor weddings, where wind and humidity could demolish a more casual hairstyle. To be comfortable in hot weather weddings, many brides choose to sweep their hair off their necks.

Dress styles can also play an equal influence in choosing a hairstyle. If your dress is heavily appliqued in the bodice, your hair can get caught or pull in the beaded areas. If you have a high, Victorian neckline, it will be complimented by a full, graceful up-do, while hair down and around the face and shoulders clutters the line. If your dress is elaborate and full, such as Princess Diana's wedding gown, a simple up-do creates a cleaner line for the face. It will focus attention on your eyes rather than on your chest and shoulders.

The Three Cs of Bridal Hair

Whatever style you choose, your hair must be cut, conditioned, and possibly colored for the wedding. One week to ten days before the wedding, your hair should be trimmed or cut. This is not the time to experiment with a new cut or a new stylist! Color should be approached equally cautiously. In the months before the wedding, you had the opportunity to try out different shades and products. Schedule coloring one week before the wedding day. To avoid a wedding-day hair disaster that will become a family legend, don't try any new coloring products or techniques. You do not want to risk an odd color or bad reaction to an untried formulation.

Conditioning should depend on the needs of your hair. If your hair tends to be oily, use a lemon juice rinse on the day before the wedding. If your hair is colored, permed, straight, or straightened, use a deep, warm cream conditioner prior to the ceremony. Because it takes an hour to get full benefits of an intense conditioning treatment, plan ahead to carve out the time for the most effective treatment. To give your hair the help it needs, try to schedule a deep conditioner at the same time your hair is colored. To avoid unexpected results, try out different conditioners, either commercially available products or the recipes that are in this book, in the months before the wedding. You need to know how your hair will react to the ingredients. Some formulations can be too thin and leave the hair dry, while richer ingredients may be too heavy and leave the hair limp.

Styling Bridal Hair

For medium-to-long hair, wedding styling is a clear departure from contemporary hair care techniques. For more than twenty-five years, loose, freshly washed hair has been the start at every beautiful look. By contrast, wedding styles usually start with day-after shampooed hair. Freshly washed hair is too slippery to hold the line of an elegant up-do.

THE WEDDING SHAMPOO

During the proceeding months, you have tried out different shampoo formulations. It is likely that your hair responds better to some more than others. Label your favorites and reserve them for the wedding day styling. When your hair is thin or tends to be oily, evaluate your hair the day after a shampoo, rather than the same-day results. If your hair seems lank and oily on the second day, keep your hair fresh with a lemon juice rinse.

WEDDING CONDITIONERS

Choose your hair care products depending on hair needs just before the wedding. You don't want a heavy conditioner that will weigh down your hair. Select one based on the status of your hair:

- ★ Frizzy: Use a silicone-based product to coat the hair.
- ★ Dull: Use a hot oil conditioner to restore shine.
- ★ Damaged: Try a deep protein conditioner.
- ★ Healthy: A light creme rinse should be massaged lightly to the body and the tips of the hair, avoiding the roots.

New Techniques

Most bridal styles start in the same way: hair is misted with a thermal-activated spray and wound on hot rollers. When the rollers are cool, the hair is sectioned, and then each piece is back-combed for texture and body. As it is positioned, it is sprayed again to hold the line. This method controls ends and edges as it retextures and reforms the hair.

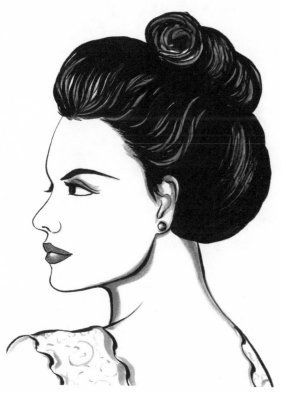

The Gibson Girl

BRIDAL CLASSIC #1: THE GIBSON GIRL

This intensely feminine style is a very soft, graceful look that requires at least medium-length hair to be properly executed. There are two ways to do the Gibson girl look. With very long hair, you can set the hair on hot rollers, remove them, and allow the hair to cool. Comb out thoroughly, and gather hair as though you were going to make a ponytail. Bend over at the waist, and turn your hair as you push it forward so you get fullness in front and looseness in back. To finish, position the chignon in the center, with the crown of the hair soft and full. For extra volume and control, hair can be slightly back-combed first to give firmer texture, rather than volume, before forming the ponytail.

For hair that is barely shoulder-length, or just to the collarbone, (1) the Gibson girl is set on medium-hot rollers, three in two rows on each side and six from the hair line to the back of the neck. (2) When the rollers are cool, separate the hair into five sections, and secure with clips. (3) Backcomb each section, smoothing the topside with a brush. Roll it into a barrel curl, positioned about two inches from the hair line. Push the hair forward to achieve desired fullness. Anchor the section with bobby pins. If your hair is thick and/or long, divide each section into three smaller strands and roll down each one to barrel curls that are secured with bobby pins. (4) Do the back section last. It can be difficult, so practice with a bridesmaid who can do it on the wedding day. The Gibson girl look works beautifully with a circlet of flowers, a tiara, or a crown at the front, and a veil at the back. It is a romantic, feminine look that works for romantic or traditional styles. It is usually worn at formal and semiformal traditional weddings, but it may be too elaborate for informal ceremonies and outdoor weddings where styles are more casual.

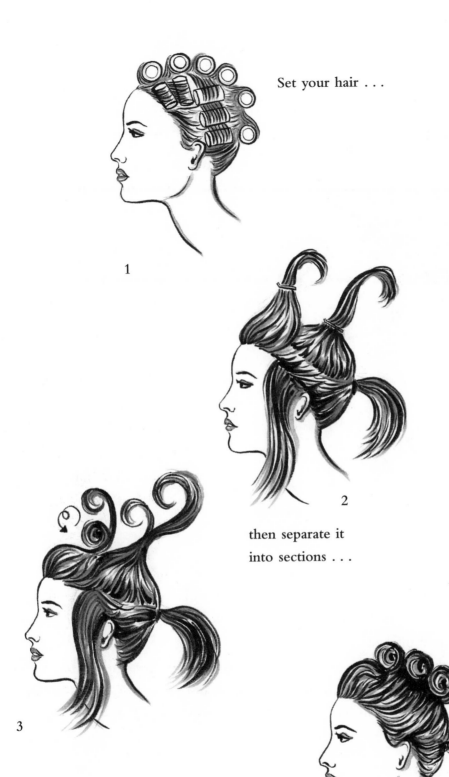

Set your hair . . .

1

2

then separate it
into sections . . .

3

and roll each section into a
barrel curl.

4

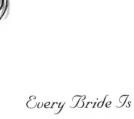

Every Bride Is
Beautiful
131

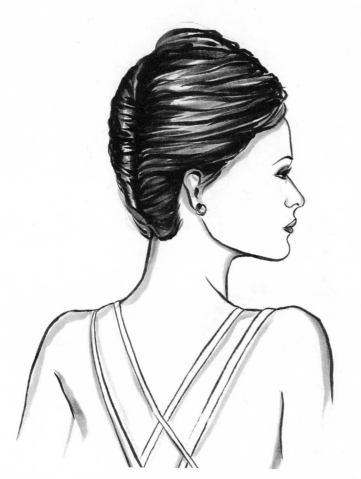

BRIDAL CLASSIC #2: THE FRENCH TWIST

There are two approaches to the French twist. For medium length, (1) backcomb your hair, smoothing the surface with a brush, and positioning it to one side. Run a line of bobby pins up the center to anchor the twist. (2) Sweep the hair back and over the bobby pins, fold it under and (3) secure it with hair pins.

With very long hair, the hair is gathered into a long, low ponytail, which actually helps your hair lose some volume. Then the hair is twisted—and gently moved upward. As the twist is laid down, it is pulled up and pinned to the scalp. The top then can be arranged in a chignon or barrel curls.

The French twist can be worn with virtually any style of dress, but it looks particularly beautiful with traditional or contemporary styles. It is a formal style, but because it was worn as a daytime look in the 1950s and 1960s, it still looks good at all weddings, from informal to ultraformal.

If properly executed, a French twist can be worn outdoors and last through a night of dancing. But if it's just twisted up and quickly pinned, gravity will alter its appearance and shape and it will start to fall.

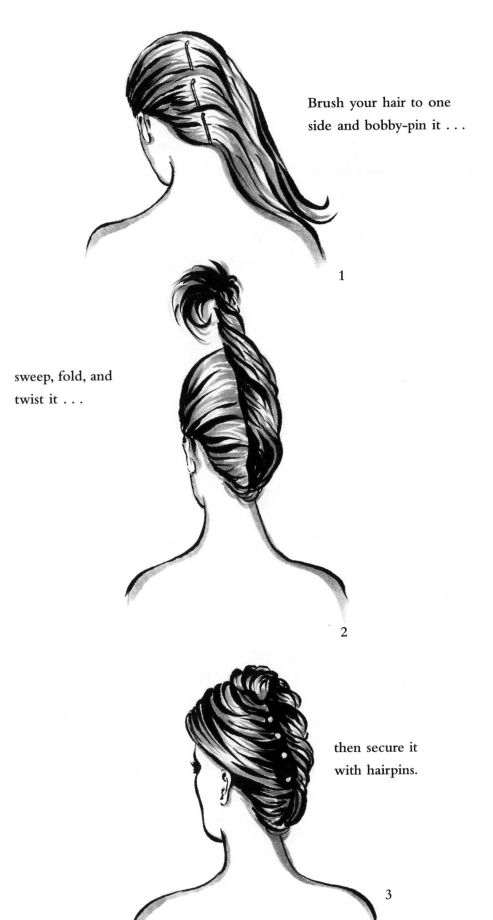

Brush your hair to one
side and bobby-pin it . . .

1

sweep, fold, and
twist it . . .

2

then secure it
with hairpins.

3

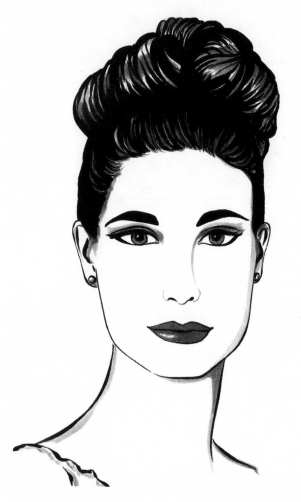

BRIDAL CLASSIC #3:
THE HIGH CHIGNON

The high chignon is one of the easiest and most attractive up-dos that can be done for both medium and long hair. For medium-length hair, the back can be twisted into a French twist. The rest of the hair is fashioned into barrel curls so that the effect is a top-knot chignon. It is particularly beautiful with a circlet of flowers around the chignon and a veil at the back. This style works beautifully with almost every type of gown. It lends itself to headpieces that go in front of the chignon, such as a crown or tiara, and also goes well with headpieces that anchor at the back, such as a bow or flower on a small comb.

The high chignon can be a simple bun done even by someone who is not good with their hair. For an elegant and simple chignon, (1) start by forming two ponytails, a thin one on top, and a fuller one underneath. (2) Wrap the smaller ponytail around the larger one to hide the rubber band, and fasten it with bobby pins. (3) The larger ponytail should be lightly backcombed, smoothed with a brush, then folded under and pinned to the head. The crown can be back-combed for soft volume or pulled tight for a smooth, modern look. Other chignon styles can feature a cluster of barrel curls, a rounded bun, or a coiled spiral. If you have a round or long face, the front can be softened with bangs.

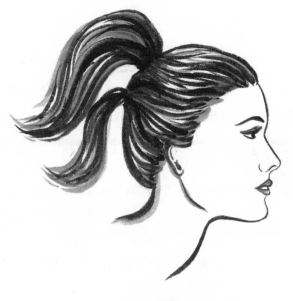

Make two ponytails . . .

1

wrap and secure them . . .

2

then fold under to
make a chignon.

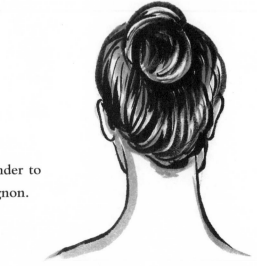

3

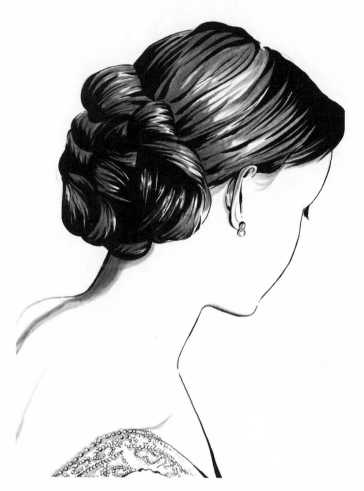

BRIDAL CLASSIC #4: THE LOW CHIGNON

The low chignon looks relatively simple but is actually difficult to execute. Your hair needs to have a certain flexibility—or you need to backcomb it carefully to control the formation of the chignon. Some stylists, such as Robert Collinge, the official hairstylist at Harrods, covers his low chignon with a very, very fine net to control the strands of hair. It is a beautiful, elegant Grecian look, but requires very long, flexible hair to form a smooth, rounded design. This was beautifully worn by Carolyn Bessette when she wed J.F.K., Jr. (1) Smooth all hair rather tightly into a ponytail. (2) Backcomb the ponytail, then smooth the surface with a paddle brush. Then (3), fold the hair under and secure it with bobby pins. Cover the chignon with a fine hair net.

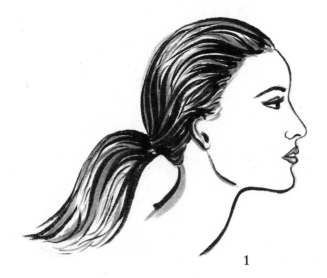

Make a ponytail . . .

1

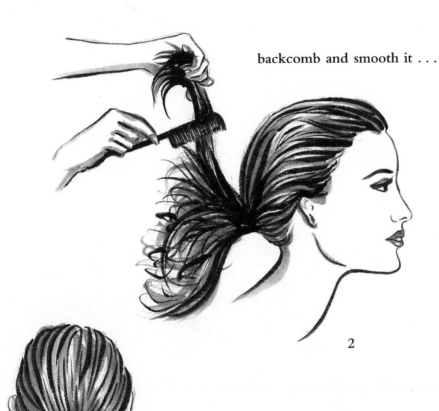

backcomb and smooth it . . .

2

then make a chignon.

3

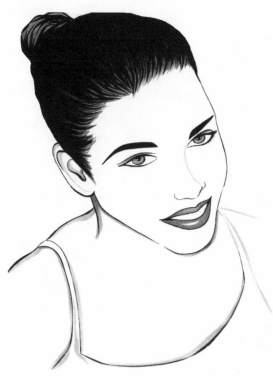

BRIDAL CLASSIC #5:
THE BALLERINA BUN

Many of the most contemporary bridal gown designers show their work with models who have hair that is simply pulled back tightly, in a simple chignon, slicked with gel, and completely covered by the veil. Bend over at the waist and **(1)** gather your hair into a tight ponytail. Twist it tightly and **(2)** coil it around itself to form a bun. **(3)** Slick back the top, sides, and back with gel to control loose strands. The ballerina bun is a very elegant, ethereal look, and looks best if your face is oval or heart-shaped. If you tend to have square or rounded cheeks, this may not provide enough softness for your facial contours. But it is certainly an extremely simple and long-lasting hairdo to execute. It can be done with medium-length hair that is simply pulled back straight in a low ponytail, and then the hair is completely covered by the veil. After the ceremony, many brides then put a bow or flowers around the ponytail so that there is decoration in the hair without the veil.

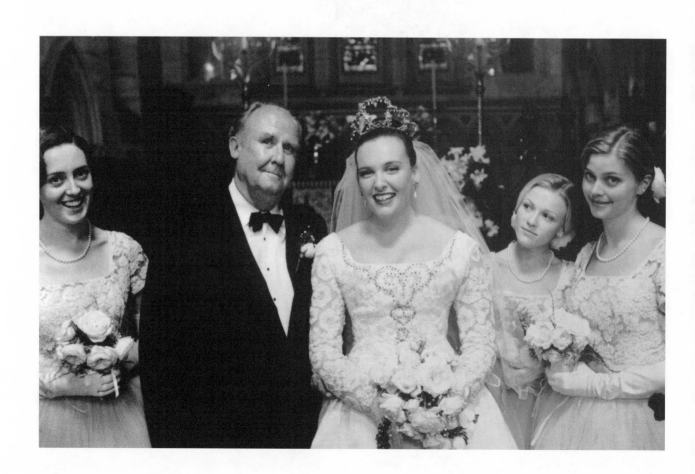

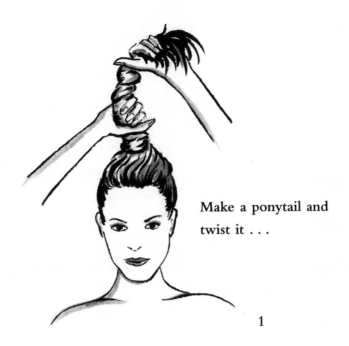

Make a ponytail and
twist it . . .

1

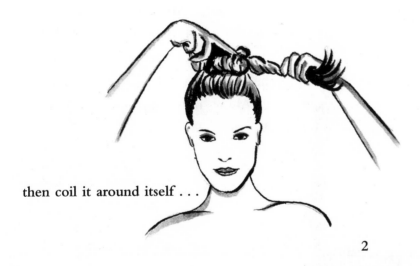

then coil it around itself . . .

2

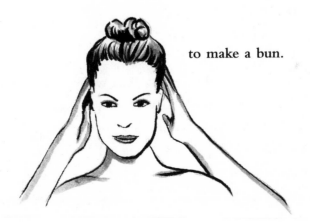

to make a bun.

3

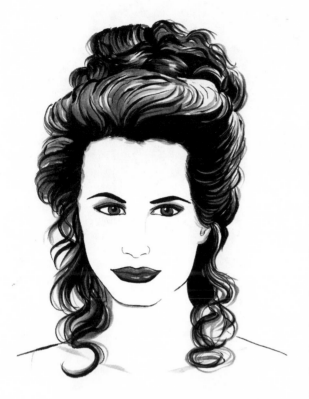

BRIDAL CLASSIC #6: THE CASCADE

One of the most elaborate of bridal styles, the cascade works best with thick hair that has a natural curve or wave. The hair should be wound on heated rollers to control the degree of curl. When the curlers are cool, brush out the hair to relax the line and (1) separate it into five sections. Divide section A into smaller sections. (2) Backcomb each part of section A and roll it into a barrel curl. Secure each curl with bobby pins. (3) Backcomb section B, smooth the surface with a brush, and anchor it to the crown of your head. Be careful to mold the hair to provide height and softness. As before, separate the strand into smaller sections, and arrange in barrel curls. Repeat the same steps with section C. (4) Section D should be lightly backcombed at the root area and rolled halfway into barrel curls. The remaining strands should be rolled around a hot curling iron for twenty seconds to form loose, spiral curls. Always mist each section with hairspray before and after rolling into curls.

---

quick tip:

The Bridal Beauty Shirt

Wear a loose white men's shirt when you get ready for your wedding day. It's easy to take on and off and will not mess up a hairdo like a T-shirt that goes over the head. The color will help the makeup artist judge what colors to use that will work with your white dress.

1

Separate
your hair
into
sections . . .

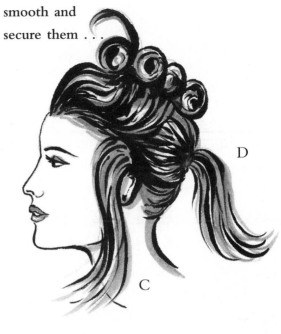

B

A

D

C

3

smooth and
secure them . . .

D

C

2

roll them into barrel
curls . . .

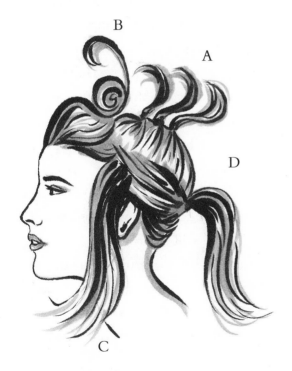

B

A

D

C

4

then curl the loose strands
with a curling iron.

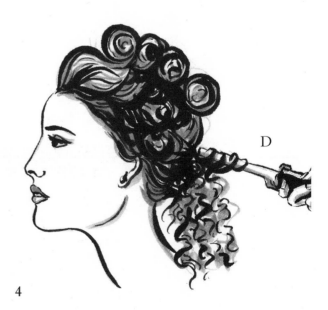

D

Choosing a Bridal Stylist

Bridal Hair Supplies

Shampoo

Conditioner

Thermal-activated hair spray

Hot rollers

Electric brush

Hair spray

Flat paddle brush

Comb

Hair pins

Bobby pins

Hair clips

Rat-tail comb

At least four months before the wedding, start exploring styling options. If you are going to have your hair professionally styled for your wedding, try out several stylists to choose the one who understands your hair and taste best. To find the person you need, ask for recommendations from your wedding consultant, photographer, or friends who have been recently married. Schedule a time for consultation and a hairstyle run-through. Bring a photo of your dress and the headpiece, if you have it. Have the hair stylist actually complete the look as if it were the wedding.

In a typical consultation, the stylist discusses the style and drapes the hair in an approximation, and there is no fee for this service. But if you want to be certain of both the hairstyle and stylist's skill, book a complete appointment, which you will have to pay for. Your hair will be washed, set, and arranged as if it were the actual wedding day. When the stylist is finished, walk around with the hairstyle, watching to see how it holds up. It gives you an opportunity to judge the quality of the stylist's work as well as to see how comfortable the style feels for you. Examine the work carefully. Is it what you had in mind? Does it stay together all day, or does it fall and straggle in a few hours? A complete run-through gives you a chance to try out your headpiece. If you've not yet purchased one, go shopping for the headpiece and veil with your wedding hairstyle.

When you find a stylist you like, make sure they are available for your wedding date. If you have a morning or afternoon wedding, they must be able to come to your house to do your hair. The hours before a daytime wedding are far too hectic to work in several hours at a hair dresser. A nighttime ceremony allows you a choice of visiting a salon or having your hair done at home. If your hair is to be done at home, discuss what supplies the stylist will need and what they will bring.

If your bridal party also wants their hair done, make sure that there are enough operators available either at the salon or who will come to your house to be able to take care of the bridal party in two hours or less. Since it takes about an hour to do each head of hair, plan on one stylist for every two to three bridal party members.

Selecting Your Personal Bridal Hairstyle

The choice of hairstyle can depend on your choice of veil and headpiece. In almost every case, brides purchase a dress and headpiece before they choose their hairstyle. Fortunately, all hair lengths and textures can be arranged into beautiful styles that accommodate a variety of headpieces. Give yourself the opportunity to try out different styles. Follow instructions for a hairdo run-through and then shop for a bridal headpiece. Take a disposable or Polaroid camera with you to see how they look in photos.

Styling the Rest of the Wedding Party

It is nice if there is a sense of unity to the bridal party. They don't have to look like Rockettes with identical hairstyles, but if you are wearing your hair up, it is nice to have all the bridesmaids wear their hair up in styles that suit their hair texture and length. They, too, should have run-throughs with a stylist before the wedding so that there is no last-minute crisis before the ceremony. If you are having the stylist come to you, make sure that there are enough supplies for everyone, including shampoos for different hair types, enough clips, bobby pins, brushes, and hair spray, as well as mirrors to give the wedding party the opportunity to take proper care of their hair.

Summary of Hairstyles and Headpieces

	HIGH CHIGNON	LOW CHIGNON	FRENCH TWIST	GIBSON	CASCADE	HALF AND HALF	DOWN
Flowers	Y	Y	Y	Y	Y	Y	Y
Bows	Y	Y	Y	Y	Y	Y	Y
Tiara	Y	Y	Y	Y	Y	Y	Y
Circlet	Y	Y	Y	Y	Y	Y	Y
Wreath	N	Y	Y	N	Y	Y	Y
Headband	N	N	N	N	N	Y	Y
Hat	N	Y	N	N	N	Y	Y
Crown	Y	N	Y	Y	N	Y	Y

Key: Y = Yes, N = No

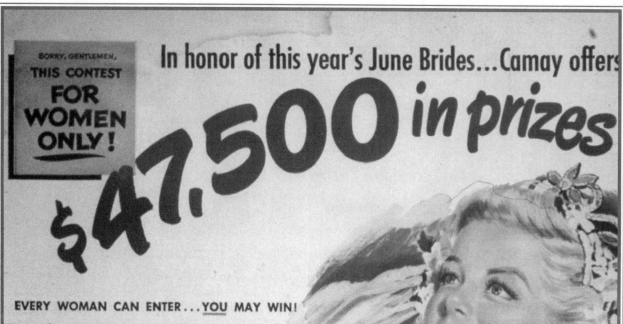
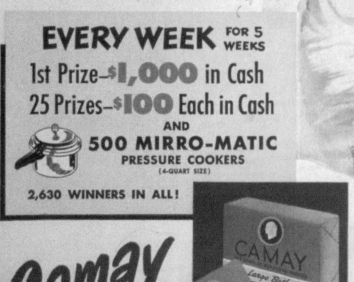

CHAPTER EIGHT

Rings on Her Fingers and Bells on Her Toes

goals:
....

* **To help nails grow strong**
* **To learn the healthiest way to manicure**
* **To select the right wedding-day nail colors**

From the moment a woman becomes engaged, her hands are on view. Each time she shows her ring, the health and beauty of her nails and hands are on display. For women who regularly take good care of their nails, it is a time to keep up the beauty of their hands. For others, it can provide the motivation to grow and maintain beautiful nails perhaps for the first time in their lives.

Bridal Nail Care 101

Nails, made of the same keratin protein that is found in hair, consist of five parts. The nail plate is the part that you see and polish. It is white in color, but looks pink because it rests on the nail bed, which is rich in blood vessels. Like skin and hair, nails need moisture to stay healthy and flexible. Household products and nail polish removers can dehydrate nails leading to cracking and peeling. Helping to restore moisture with creams and lotions will prevent breakage and promote length.

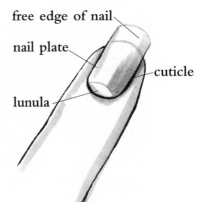

The part of the nail that grows over the fingertip is known as the free edge, and this is the part of the nail that you file. The lunula is the white half moon at the base of the nail. The nail base and matrix lying under the lunula is the source of new nail growth. Poor health, bad nutrition, or a blow to the matrix can disrupt nail growth. Enclosing the nail plate is the

145

The Duchess of Windsor

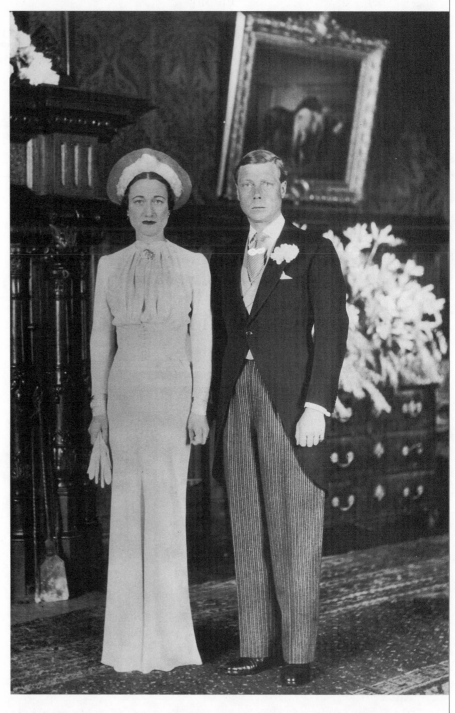

When American divorcée Wallis Simpson married the Duke of Windsor, she needed a wedding ensemble that would balance her personal style with the unparalleled political upheavals that her marriage would produce. She asked Mainbocher for a gown that would be consistent with her chic simplicity and that would set off her spectacular jewels, a look that would be regal rather than festive. Her long "Wallis" blue gown and matching jacket was draped into a heart shape at the bust. On her head she wore a blue straw bonnet by the legendary French milliner, Caroline Reboux. Mrs. Simpson was rather proud of her rail-thin shape, but she hated her hands, so she ordered a pair of matching blue crepe wrist-length gloves. The third finger of the left hand opened up, so that she would not need to remove her gloves when the Duke placed a platinum ring on her hand during the ceremony. The gown, which is now in the costume collection of the Metropolitan Museum of Art, established a style for second weddings that has remained in fashion for more than half a century.

cuticle, designed to keep and protect the matrix from dirt and infection. The cuticle can be pushed back, but should never be cut during a manicure. On average, the nail grows about an eighth of an inch a month, with faster growth in warm weather and slower growth as we age.

The Top Thirteen Nail Problems

With a beautiful ring on the third finger of a left hand, a bride wants beautiful, healthy nails and soft, clear hands. Despite the very best intentions, many women find it hard to achieve the look they seek. Their nails seem to peel, break, and turn yellow, and the cuticles become ragged. Fortunately, with a little time and attention, most nail problems can be easily handled at home. The first step is discovering the cause. The color and nail condition will provide necessary clues to the diagnosis of the problem.

PROBLEM #1: YELLOWED NAILS

Yellow nails are usually the result of staining from nicotine (smoking), dark nail polish, or hair dyes. To restore nails to their natural pale color, bleach the nail plate with bleach or hydrogen peroxide. Wrap an orange stick with cotton, dip in bleach, and apply to the surface and underside of the nail. Allow solution to evaporate—usually it takes less than a minute—then rinse off.

PROBLEM #2: BLUISH NAILS

Bluish nails can appear due to injury, severe stress, or chemical exposure. Best treatment is to allow the discoloration to grow out, or use an opaque polish.

PROBLEM #3: GREENISH NAILS

Greenish nails indicate mold or fungus. This can develop when separation appears between a natural and artificial nail, or wrap. The artificial covering should be removed, washed, and dried and the nail treated with a nonprescription antibiotic cream twice a day. Do not replace the artificial nail until the entire nail has grown out and healed.

PROBLEM #4: BLACK-AND-WHITE SPOTS

Black-and-white spots are usually signs of injuries or chronic illness, but they can appear for no reason at all. The best solution is to use an opaque rather than sheer polish and let the spots grow out naturally.

PROBLEM #5: HORIZONTAL RIDGES

Ridges result from an injury, such as hitting yourself with a hammer, or a too vigorous manicure. Ridge filler base coats can help smooth the surface so the manicure looks beautiful.

PROBLEM #6: BRITTLE NAILS

Brittleness is the result of exposure to detergents, irritating chemicals, or overuse of cuticle softeners. In some cases, it is hereditary. The best treatment is to use strong moisturizers, such as those containing alpha-hydroxy acids, to make sure that the water level is high in your skin. It will take six to eight months of treatment and attention to restore moisture to the nails, and you should use the nail intensive treatments on page 151.

PROBLEM #7: THIN NAILS

Thin, soft nails can be a sign of poor nutrition such as occurs with crash diets. If this happens, be sure to take a multivitamin pill and use fabric-fortified nail hardeners. Do not use nail hardeners with formaldehyde because these products tend to cause allergic reactions.

PROBLEM #8: PITTING

Pitting can be a sign of psoriasis. This is best treated by a physician and can be helped with a cortisone cream.

PROBLEM #9: GROOVES IN THE NAILS

Grooves, which are deeper than ridges, usually start at the cuticle and indicate real damage to the nail bed. They can be caused by stress, alcohol abuse, or pregnancy. These are best handled by medical treatment for underlying causes. They can be disguised with an opaque polish applied over ridge filler base coats. But you need to find out what is causing the problems in the first place.

PROBLEM #10: SPOON-SHAPED NAILS

This condition, in which nails seem to turn upward, can be caused by strong soaps or iron deficiency. It can be hereditary. (The iron deficiency can be a problem for vegetarians.)

PROBLEM #11: CLAW-SHAPED NAILS

This condition, in which nails turn down, is unattractive but not serious. Usually the result of an injury to the nail bed, the nail should be allowed to grow out to a healthy, attractive shape. Keep your nails short to minimize the down-turned tendencies.

PROBLEM #12: CRACKED NAILS

Cracked nails are often a sign of overuse of nail polish remover and dishwashing detergents. Maintain a weekly series of deep nail conditioners until the nails stop cracking.

PROBLEM #13: SEPARATION FROM THE NAIL BED

Separation from the nail bed is due to injury, allergy, drug reaction, or a response to formaldehyde. The nail needs to be grown out to heal the matrix. It is best not to use any product on these nails until the entire nail is healthy and firmly fixed to the finger.

Artificial Nails

There are two basic choices for artificial nails—sculpted and bonded—and they both are best done by professionals. Sculpted nails build up a layer of acrylic plastic over an acetate tip glued to the natural nails. The nails are sealed, shaped, and polished as usual. They can look even better than natural nails because polish never chips off the acrylic as it does off the natural nail plate. Nails will continue to grow under the sculpted nails, but the

If a nail breaks, especially right before a wedding, it can be easily fixed with a tube of nail glue and a small piece of unused paper from a tea bag.

1. Remove polish from the broken nail.
2. Apply a drop of glue to the nail break.
3. Quickly position a small bit of paper to glue before it dries.
4. Apply a drop of glue over the paper.
5. Allow glue to dry.
6. File excess paper so that you cannot see or feel the edges.
7. Apply another drop of glue and let it dry.
8. Smooth again with buffing disc until surface is smooth.
9. Reapply ridge nail filler, base coat, nail color, and top coat as in standard manicure.

acrylic layers should be removed every six weeks to give your own nails a chance to rest and breathe. This vacation would also be a good opportunity to give your nails a series of deep-conditioning treatments to restore water and flexibility. If you keep sculptured nails on too long, your natural nails will become soft, brown, and extremely unattractive.

Bonded nails are treated with acrylic gels and placed under ultraviolet lights, which bonds the gel. They too should be removed every six weeks to keep the nails strong and healthy.

Nail Care Intensive Program

The months before the wedding are a wonderful time to grow and condition your nails and care for your hands. We subject both our hands and nails to constant abuse. They're dunked in soap suds, dried out with dust and paper, seared by the sun, and buried in garden dirt. Hands and nails don't take kindly to this treatment. They rebel with dryness, chapping, red spots, redness, brown spots, and roughness and the nails become brittle, cracked, thin, and discolored.

With a regular manicure and a schedule of deep-conditioning treatments, you can restore the health and beauty to your hands and nails and maintain it easily. Every seven to ten days nails should be given a complete manicure. More frequent manicures will subject them to too much drying and manipulation. If you let too much time elapse between manicures, your nails will become chipped and dull. Not only will this look unattractive, but the nail polish itself actually strengthens and protects the nail. Every three weeks take the time to give yourself a deep-conditioning treatment. Vary the treatments you use to provide the greatest improvement.

The Basic Manicure

1. Remove polish with a cotton ball.
2. Rinse off and dry thoroughly.
3. File the nails gently in one direction.
4. Apply cuticle cream or softener and massage in.
5. Soak nails in warm water enriched with a drop of shampoo for no more than four or five minutes.
6. Scrub nails gently with a soft toothbrush.
7. Push back cuticle gently with a moonstone stick.
8. Snip dry cuticles with clippers, being careful not to open the cuticle seal.
9. Clean hands and nails under and around the cuticles with a cotton-tipped orange stick that has been dipped in polish remover.
10. Buff nails to improve circulation. Be sure to lift chamois each time you buff to avoid overheating.
11. Apply base coat with ridge filler or fiber hardeners and allow to dry.
12. Apply one coat of polish and allow to dry.
13. Apply top coat and allow to dry.
14. Dry for 15 minutes in the air, away from heat or fans, which can cause bubbling.
15. Apply quick dry with a brush, rather than use an aerosol, which can dry out the nail and dull the polish.

HAND AND NAIL CONDITIONING TREATMENTS

Warm Tuscan Rub

This warm oil treatment softens hands and cuticles.

1. Heat olive oil for eight seconds in microwave.
2. Massage into cuticles.
3. Slip each hand into a small plastic bag.
4. Rest for ten minutes.
5. Remove plastic bags and wash hands with rich superfatted soap. Rinse and dry thoroughly.

Russian Cuticle Softener

The lactic acid in the yogurt softens hardened cuticles, and the wheat germ rubs them away.

1. Combine 3 tablespoons of whole milk yogurt, 1 teaspoon wheat germ oil, and 1 drop of spirits of peppermint.
2. Combine all ingredients in a bowl.
3. Rub mixture into cuticles.
4. Rest hands for twenty minutes on a clean towel.
5. Wash off with superfatted soap, rubbing cuticles with dry washcloth.

Beechnut Night Cream

The fruit acids in the applesauce lift the dry, dead skin cells as the Crisco moisturizes the surface.

1. Melt 3 tablespoons of Crisco over low heat; beat in 1 tablespoon of baby applesauce until mixture is creamy.
2. Dissolve 1 teaspoon of borax into mixture.
3. Remove from heat, pour mixture into a clean container and store in refrigerator for up to one week.
4. To use, take out 1 tablespoon of the mixture and rub it well into your hands before going to bed.

Grape Nail Soak

The yogurt and grapes provide two different types of fruit acids to soften and strengthen the nails.

1. Combine 3 tablespoons of yogurt, a quarter cup seedless grapes, crushed, 1 teaspoon of glycerin, and 1 teaspoon of peach kernel oil.
2. Rub mixture into hands and nails.
3. Cover each hand with a plastic bag.
4. Rest for twenty minutes.
5. Wash hands with superfatted soap and dry nails thoroughly.

Napa Valley Hand and Nail Mask

The egg yolk and olive oil create a face mask for the hands.

1. Combine 1 beaten egg, 1 tablespoon white wine, and 1 teaspoon olive oil.
2. Massage mixture into hands and wrap in warm wash towels. Enclose hands in a large plastic bag.
3. Rest for twenty minutes.
4. Wash with superfatted soap and dry thoroughly.

NAIL CARE NECESSITIES

Nail care products are beauty care's biggest bargain. You can assemble a collection of the best tools, lotions, and lacquers for less than the cost of a single bottle of high-powered moisturizer. Put together a kit of products that you will use at home or take to a professional manicurist.

Emery Boards:
You will need two types, a thick, black board to shape nails and a round buffing disc to smooth the rough edges.

Polish Remover:
This essential nail care element can be the most damaging. The least drying formulations are acetone-free.

Cuticle Softeners:
These softeners dissolve dry, dead cuticle skin without damaging the important cuticle seal. Best new formulations include alpha-hydroxy acids.

Liquid Fiber Base Coat:
This wonderful product serves a dual purpose. It strengthens weak or brittle nails and protects them from becoming stained from dark-colored polishes.

Top Coat:
These are thinner than the polish or the base coat and they are meant to give a thickness and greater resistance to abrasion and maintain a gloss.

Chamois cloth is used to bring a natural shine.

Nail Glue:

A strong, fast-acting adhesive, nail glue is designed to be easy on nails and skin. All-purpose household quick glues are much too strong and irritating to use on the body.

Orange Sticks:

Orange sticks are used for cleaning under the nails and for controlling the cuticles.

Vitamin E Capsules:

400 mg capsules are snipped open with a nail clipper and massaged into the cuticles.

Nail Clippers:

The most expensive manicure item in your box. You want a sharp, pointed instrument that will accurately remove tiny bits of skin that should come off without touching the cuticle seal, which should remain closed.

Quick-Dry Oil:

Use the brush-on rather than spray-on formulations, which tend to dull polish shine.

Bridal Nail Care Shopping List

* Nail brush
* Orange stick
* Cuticle remover
* Pumice stone
* Cotton pads
* Toenail clippers
* Cuticle clippers
* Ridge filler base coat
* Sheer polish
* Quick-dry oil
* Top coat
* Almond oil
* Toe separator
* Vitamin E capsules
* Rich hand lotion
* Polish remover
* Blue nail polish

The Other Ten Nails

Not as visible as the hands, the feet and toenails still need attention. Many wedding shoes are open and airy, exposing long-hidden heels while sun-soaked honeymoons bare toes and soles. While hands take at least a month to get into shape, a single pedicure can transform your feet. Two nights before your wedding, set aside time to do a complete pedicure.

The Wedding Pedicure

1. Soak feet in warm water enriched with a few drops of almond oil for 15 minutes.
2. Slough hard heel skin with a pumice stone.
3. Dry feet thoroughly with a towel.
4. Smooth cuticle cream on toes and push cuticles back with an orange stick.
5. Snip off loose dry skin with cuticle clippers.
6. Rinse off feet with lukewarm water.
7. Cut toenails straight across to avoid ingrown nails.
8. File away rough edges.
9. Massage feet with rich lotion.
10. Clean off toes with cotton-tipped orange stick dipped in polish remover. Clean under and top of nails with the same orange stick.
11. Slip on toe separator.
12. Apply base coat.
13. Apply blue toenail polish (as in "something old, something new").
14. Apply top coat.
15. Sit quietly for 20 minutes to give nails time to dry thoroughly.

If you have been following the wedding hand care program for the four months before your wedding, your nails should be strong and well-shaped. Plan to manicure your nails the day before the wedding. Done earlier, nails may chip and dull, while on the day of the ceremony life is too hectic to take the hour you need to shape, polish, and properly dry your nails.

Wedding Nail Styles

The most beautiful wedding nails are pale—almost sheer—in a length that ranges from short (the free edge reaches just to the tip of the fingertip), average (the free edge extends a quarter inch over the tip), and long (up to a half inch from the tip of the finger). In an era when women work with their hands and intellect, long curved talons are relics of another era.

Your choice of color depends both on your complexion and your dress. Warm skin tones work best with creamy, ivory shades, while cool skin tones look best in white colors. Sheer pink works

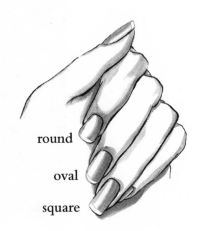

round

oval

square

well on everyone except those with ruddy complexions. Nails can be worn naturally or with a thin, white tip of a French manicure. Try out different shades of polish at cosmetic counters in the weeks and months before your wedding. If several colors seem to work, do one hand in each color before you go for a fitting of your gown to see which shade works best with the color and fabric of your dress.

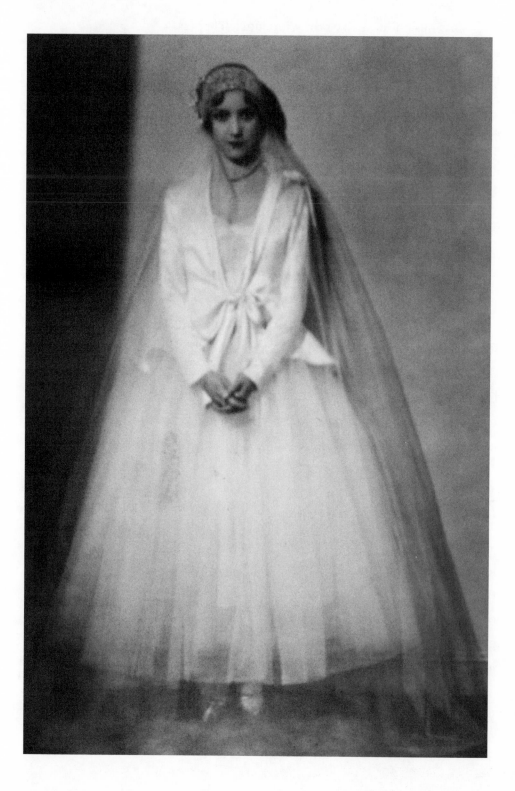

One week before the wedding, treat your hands to a softening mask.

1. Mix together 1 egg yolk, 1 tablespoon of honey, 1 tablespoon of oatmeal, and 1 tablespoon of wheat germ.
2. Massage the mixture into your hands and nails.
3. Put hands in a small plastic bag and wrap in hot towels.
4. Keep mask on for 20 minutes.
5. Rinse off with lukewarm water and manicure as usual.

The day before the wedding, set out a quiet hour for a careful manicure.

1. Soak a cotton ball with polish remover and stroke it against the nail, avoiding the cuticle. Polish will dry it out.
2. Wash off the remover but don't soak the nails, since you will be shaping them with a file.
3. File with a black emery board going in just one direction.
4. Snip off the end of a capsule of vitamin E and rub it into the cuticles.
5. Massage hand lotion into the cuticles as well as the palms and tops of the hands.
6. Slip hands in plastic bag and relax for five minutes.
7. Remove plastic bag and soak hands in warm water with a drop of liquid soap.
8. With a soft toothbrush, gently scrub nails and skin on the hand.
9. Rub a fine pumice stone along the rough sides of the fingers.
10. Smooth buffing disk on the nails.
11. Gently push back the cuticles with a cotton-tipped orange stick.
12. Cut loose, dry skin on the edges of the fingernails, but avoid cutting the cuticles at the base of the nails.
13. Clean under the nails with a cotton-tipped orange stick soaked in soapy water.
14. If the nails look yellow, dip a cotton-tipped orange stick in hydrogen peroxide and gently rub on top of and under the nail, rinse off, and dry thoroughly.
15. Buff nails to a smooth surface. It will give a healthy glow that looks wonderful under a sheer, pale polish. Lift chamois after each stroke to avoid overheating.
16. Line up polish, top coat, and base coat in front of you and loosen the tops. Starting with your pinky finger, apply liquid fiber base coat. If

your nails are very weak, apply one coat vertically, allow to dry for 60 seconds, then apply another coat horizontally and dry for another 60 seconds.

17. Pull out brush from bottle of polish and remove excess from brush before stroking it on nail.

18. Starting with the pinky, stroke the center then each side, moving from base to tip in a quick, smooth motion. Use only one coat of polish to produce a sheer, delicate color.

19. Let nails dry another 60 seconds, then apply the top coat to add shine and prevent chipping. Let nails air-dry for 10 minutes to avoid bubbling.

20. With a tiny paint brush, apply baby oil on or around the nails. Avoid aerosol quick-dry products, which dull the finish.

21. Try not to use your hands for the next hour.

The French Bridal Manicure

1. Go through steps one through fourteen of the traditional manicure (p. 157).

2. With a good-quality eyeliner brush, apply a pale pink, beige, white, or ivory opaque polish to the curve of the free edge of the nail.

3. Dry for 2 to 3 minutes.

4. Apply a coat of sheer beige or pink transparent color over the entire nail.

5. Allow to dry for 4 minutes.

6. Apply another coat of polish.

7. Dry for 2 minutes.

8. Cover with a top coat and allow to dry for 10 minutes.

9. Apply a quick-dry oil.

The Wartime Bride

Without time to catch its collective breath, the world plunged from the Depression of the 1930s into World War II. Strict rationing of food and fabric during wartime led to innovative wedding choices. Brides were encouraged to marry their military grooms in simple street clothes rather than a wedding gown, a choice that was seen as both patriotic to her country and an expression of love to her soldier husband. Friends and family frequently donated food ration points for a festive wartime wedding dinner.

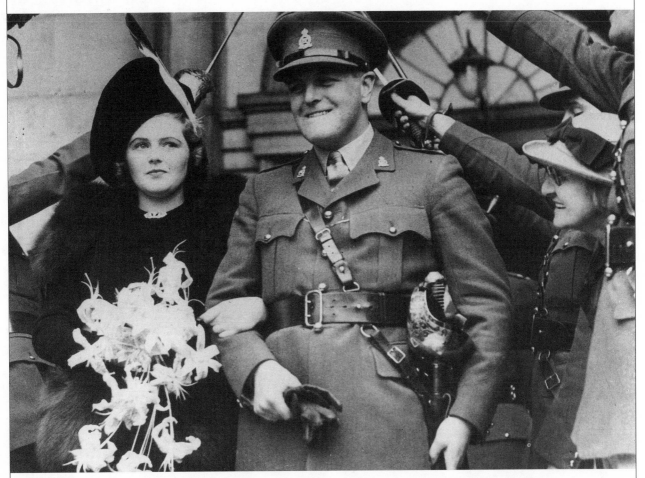

Makeup was in equally short supply. Most factory machines had been requisitioned for the war effort—for example, the manufacturing equipment for lipstick cases was retooled to produce bullets. Even the cardboard boxes and cellophane wrapping of beauty products were directed to military needs. Ever resourceful, wartime brides came up with imaginative solutions. They made rouge water by soaking red ribbon and rose petals in wine, brushed on boot black as mascara, and stroked on brown shoe polish to darken eyebrows. Nail polish was particularly hard to buy since the basic ingredients were used in explosive devices. To groom their nails, the wartime bride buffed her nails with a suede cloth to a sheer pink, shiny finish.

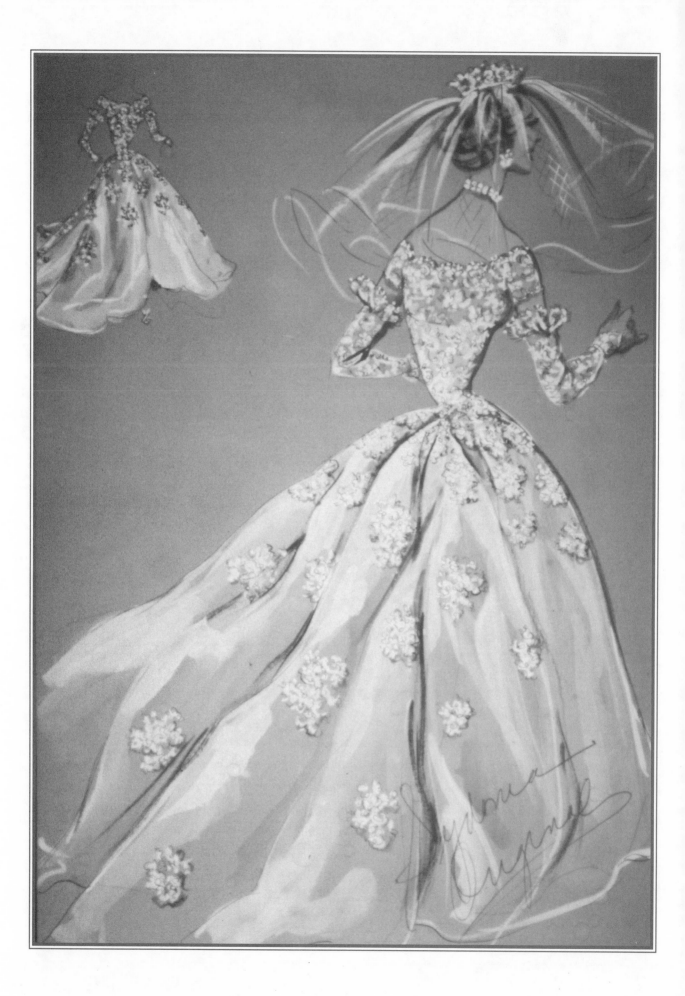

CHAPTER NINE

Questions and Answers

Q: Where can I find hair stylists and makeup artists who are experienced in bridal beauty?

Start to search for a stylist by asking friends and family for recommendations from people they have used for their weddings. You can see firsthand how they work, the quality of their work, and hear what working with them is like. If you haven't recently been involved in weddings or if you're the first one or the last one in your group to get married, your local bridal salon can refer you to people who are experienced in the field. Your wedding consultant, your bridal salon, or even the function hall where you are having your wedding likely will be able to give you the name and number of a skilled stylist in your area. In February and June, there's a lot of media attention paid to weddings and often bridal stylists will be profiled on TV and the press or will run advertisements in the local paper.

Q: I never wear makeup. Do I have to wear it at my wedding?

This is a very common question today, because a lot of women don't wear makeup. And the answer is, it is your wedding and you have to be comfortable. On the other hand, you want to look and feel beautiful in person as well as in the pictures. The type of makeup that bothers most non-makeup wearers is the sensation of foundation on the face. If you have good, clear skin, you can get away with a very light dusting of powder or a lightly tinted moisturizer. That, plus a little mascara on your eyelashes and a light lip gloss on your lips, will give you the little bit of polish that is really necessary. If you really hate the sensation of makeup, try to avoid a formal wedding, where a bare face with a formal hairstyle and dress will not give you as luminous a look as you would like. However, if you have a sun-soaked beachside wedding, a light tan and a little lip gloss is all that you should be expected to wear.

Q: Should all the bridesmaids have the same hairstyle?

They don't need to look like Rockettes, with everybody having the same hairstyle, but it's nice to have a unity to the bridal party. It is nice, for example, for all the bridesmaids to wear their hair in an up-do. They can wear it in different styles to flatter their faces and hair length, but it gives a continuity without a cookie-cutter appearance.

Q: I work with my hands, and they're a mess.
Wouldn't a manicure call attention to them?

A manicure actually helps your hands and nails get into shape. Don't wait until the day before the wedding for your first manicure. You should try to get your hands into as good a shape as possible during the prewedding period with regular manicures to help the nails grow, get cuticles under control, and create a finished, polished look.

Q: What should I decide on first? My bridal hairstyle or my headpiece?

Most headpieces can work with a range of bridal hairstyles, and you are also going to be limited by the length and texture of your hair as to what hairstyle you choose. It would be a good idea to think about how you want to wear your hair and then try on different headpieces that go with that. For example, if you want to wear your hair up in a French twist, you will see that a crown or tiara or back treatment will work beautifully but that a hat, headband, or even a wreath can be a problem. You don't have to make the final decision when you buy the headpiece, but you should have a general idea of what hairstyle you'd like to wear.

Q: Should the hair stylist and makeup artist come to me
or should the work be done in their shop?

That depends a great deal on where you live and the time of your wedding. Morning weddings or even noontime weddings need a stylist and

The 1950s Bride

···

The opulent lace-and-silk gowns of the 1950s were a visible symbol of postwar celebration and prosperity. Wedding gowns were bigger and more elaborate than they had been for more than fifty years. Bridal makeup started with a rather thick flesh-toned foundation to create a flawless rather than pale complexion. Cake rouge added cheek color while turquoise eye shadow and black eyeliner defined a bride's eyes. Often the bride chose red lipstick to match her long red nails. The fairytale white dress combined with strong heavy makeup created a look that was both innocent and erotic.

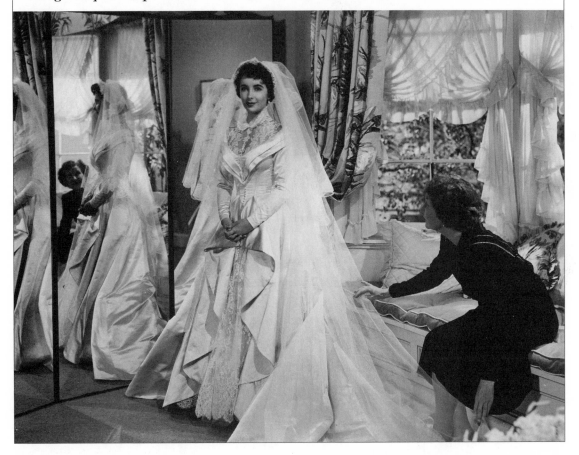

makeup artist who will come to your house. If you live out of town, it is really much more convenient to have them come to you. However, if you're having a nighttime wedding and you live in a city—and it's fairly easy for you to get to the stylist—you might find it easier and actually less stressful to get out of your house for a while to get your hair and makeup done. Be sure when you go that you wear a blouse shirt that buttons up the front so that you don't have to worry about pulling the shirt over your head, which will disrupt the hairstyle and makeup.

Q: *What can I do to frizz-proof my hair during a humid summer wedding?*

After shampooing, use a creme rinse to relax the hair and a silicone-based gel to provide a raincoat-like protection against humidity.

Q: *Should my bridesmaids wear the same nail polish?*

The same color nail polish is a very nice touch for all bridesmaids and it's certainly not an imposition on their own personal style to do that. It creates unity and continuity, and it looks glaring if one person is in dark red and another person is in a pale color, particularly in wedding photographs.

Q: *My back tends to break out. What kind of makeup can cover it?*

I think before you talk about covering back breakout problems, you should try to control it. One of the leading causes of back blemishes is long hair; the oils get on the back and provoke breakouts. The best way to deal with this is to take the hair off your back and then to apply drying lotions to the back. If your back has a problem, avoid backless dresses that will just reveal problems, especially if stress produces even more breakouts on your wedding day.

Q: *I plan to lose twenty pounds for my wedding.*
Should I wait to lose weight before looking for a dress?*

Twenty pounds is a large weight loss to anticipate. Unless your wedding is more than a year off, this is asking a lot of your body, especially if weight control has always been a problem. I would wait to lose at least ten pounds before shopping for the wedding dress. This isn't going to significantly change the style of dress that you're going to wear, but it will certainly change the fit of whatever gown you choose. If you wait until you lose the weight, you may wait so long that you won't be able to get a wedding dress in time.

Q: *Can I wear a veil with a short dress?*

You can wear a short, shoulder-length veil with a short dress, but if it is a second wedding, it is usually more appropriate to wear a hat or headpiece without a veil.

Q: I'm a nurse, and I wash my hands frequently, so they're always chapped and lotions don't seem to help. I want to show off my ring, but my hands are so red and chapped.

Try switching to a soap with antibacterial moisturizing gel rather than bar soap. You will get the same antibacterial action but without the drying factor. Try to apply an alpha-hydroxy moisturizer each time that you wash your hands. Apply a double layer of hand lotion at night. Put one layer on, let it absorb, and then add another.

Q: I wear eyeglasses, I really can't see without them, and I don't like contacts. Can I wear them during my wedding?

According to wedding planner Marcy Blum, eyeglasses and wedding attire have an uneasy relationship. "If a bride does not feel comfortable without her glasses, it is important to wear her hair off the face to avoid above-the-neck clutter. The veil should be on a comb rather than attached to a headpiece, which would compete for attention with the eyeglasses."

Q: When should the dress be fitted?

According to Monica Hickey, the final fitting should be no more than one month before the wedding. "Brides tend to go up and down in weight in the months before the wedding," she explained. "If the dress is fitted too far in advance, it may require unnecessary adjustments."

Q: My sister developed a huge cyst on her chin two days before her wedding. We have the same skin type, and I'm terrified it will happen to me. What can I do?

If this happens, go to your dermatologist, who will give you a cortisone shot right in the center of the cyst. This often reduces inflammation without creating a lump or redness.

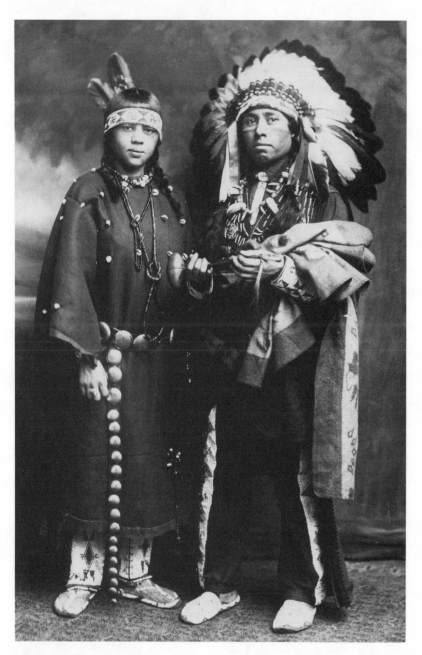

Nineteenth-century Native-American bride and groom.

Q: Should the mothers of the bride and the groom wear the same length and style of dress?

It will look better if the mothers of the bride and groom have a compatible look. It does look odd if the mother of the bride is in a short dress and the mother of the groom is in a long dress. Traditionally it is the bride's mother who chooses the style. Be prepared; this could cause problems to flare up between the new in-laws. If the groom's mother protests, offer to pay for the dress so that she doesn't feel she's being forced to buy a dress she hates.

Q: I have a child, but I was never married. Can I still wear a white wedding gown?

According to etiquette, you should probably wear an off-white or creamy dress, or perhaps one with a pale pastel tint to it.

Q: Should I wear white nail polish?

Opaque, white nail polish does not create enough contrast between the nails and the dress and tends to look odd. You're better off with a pale pink or a sheer nail polish.

Q: I always look better with a tan. Can I get one before the wedding?

A tan tends to look greasy and sweaty in photographs, so unless you're having a beachside wedding, leave the tanning for the honeymoon.

Q: I got a permanent wave that has made my hair look frizzy. Can I now use a straightener to smooth it out?

No, don't even think about it. Your hair is already damaged from the perm. Adding a straightener can cause terrible breakage and hair loss. To relax an over-frizzy perm, try deep, intensive conditioners for several weeks and then use an electric comb to give it increased softness.

Q: I want to be a pale blond bride, but when I color my hair, I always wind up as a strawberry blond. What can I do?

There could be two things working here. The first is that your lightener could not be strong enough to lift the existing color from your hair, or it's not left on long enough. The result? You're going to end up with red tones. To figure out the problem, cut a small strand of hair from the back of your head and test it with different bleaching times with the products that you are using. If you are leaving the hair-coloring cream on for the maximum time, but still produce red tones, you need a stronger formulation. Check the color tones on the box to judge if you are confusing the hair color of the model with the actual lightening potential of the formulation.

Q: After I lightened my hair, it looked oily but limp. How can I bring back body and color? How can I have both body and color?

Lightening treatments damage the hair somewhat, and it loses a degree of flexibility, but oil gland production has not been affected. If you are using shampoo and conditioner for chemically treated hair, the formulation may be too rich for your natural oil levels. To restore flexibility to your hair, use low-pH shampoos to strengthen the hair strand and a protein-based intensive conditioner just at the lower half of the hair strand.

Q: I don't want to change my hair color but I want something to liven it up. What should I do?

Try highlights or lowlights around your face to add a little brightness and color. If you don't like it, it will grow out in three to four months; it will not require upkeep.

Q: I'm only five feet two and am planning a formal wedding. Most of the trains are so long and heavy I look like I'm playing dress-up or pulling a plow. What style can I wear to go with my height and the formality of the event?

To add height to your frame, look for Princess-styled dresses that have enough grandeur for a formal wedding but will not give you the height-cutting effect of a bouffant ball gown wedding dress. You can use a chapel-length train that can be detached after the wedding. To increase the formality of the dress, look for embellishments of embroidery, rhinestones, or pearls, but choose a lighter fabric that will not increase the weight of the dress. Your veil should be no longer than fingertip-length and should flow to the back of your head rather than in front, which would cut your line and make you look more petite.

Q: My face has small numerous colorless bumps under the skin. Sometimes they blossom into small blemishes but mostly they just make my skin look lumpy. What can I do?

This is a classic dry skin acne, which is often caused by the use of inadequate cleaners, overuse of moisturizers, or oily sunscreens. The best treatment uses alpha-hydroxy peels or Retin-A to take off the dead cells that are clogging pores and allow the pores literally to empty themselves. It will take about two to three weeks for this to be effective.

Q: I want to wear my hair half-and-half—sides up and back down— but the barrette that I use looks ugly and lumpy behind my headpiece. How can I fix this?

Instead of using a barrette, comb up the front and sides of the hair and then anchor the sides with two bobby pins pinned at cross angles. Spray carefully: the sides will stay up and then you'll be able to place your headpiece invisibly over the bobby pins.

Q: My wedding shoes are beautiful but not that comfortable. Is it okay to change to lace-and-pearl decorated wedding sneakers for the party?

It really depends on the height of your wedding shoes. If you have high heel wedding shoes and a floor-length dress, you're going to be stepping all over your dress and veil if you change to lower shoes. If your wedding shoes are that uncomfortable, you probably have the wrong wedding shoes. However, if you have fairly low shoes to begin with and your dress is only ankle-length or above, then changing to wedding sneakers is not going to cause that much of a trampling problem.

Q: My husband wants his sister to be a bridesmaid. I have nothing against her, but she wears a nose ring and has four studs in a single ear lobe. She says she can't take them off because they will close up. But I can't bear the idea of a bridesmaid with a nose ring at a formal wedding.

It's doubtful that in the twelve-hour period of the wedding that the nose ring or the ear holes are going to close up. You can offer to pay for repiercing if they do. But it is your wedding, and if the idea of a nose ring creates a problem for you, it's something you have a right to complain about.

Q: I love my sisters-in-law and was a bridesmaid at their weddings when I was a teenager. But now they both weigh 250 pounds and have thinning gray hair. I shudder at the thought of wedding portraits flanked by two kind but huge bridesmaids.

There are bridesmaids dresses up to size 36, but it would make quite a statement to have both bridesmaids very large and older attendants. You might consider an informal wedding and have only your best friend or sister as the only attendant. Alternatively you can elect to have only children as attendants like at the marriage of Lady Diana and Prince Charles. Perhaps your sisters and sisters-in-law have sons and daughters. It's a charming look and it gets around the problem of the appearance of older bridesmaids.

Q: I'm going to wear open-toed, high-heeled sandals. Can I still wear blue nail polish on my toes?

If you have an informal wedding, this probably wouldn't be too much of a problem, but your best bet is to use something other than blue toenail polish. During the wedding the focus should be on your face and not on your feet.

Q: *I have trouble keeping my weight up, and I feel that when I try on my gown for the fitting, it is going to be too big.*

For the very small number of women who have trouble keeping on weight, you can choose a gown that requires you to be bone-slim to wear it beautifully. A gown completely beaded or made of lace or embroidery adds weight and bulk to a very thin frame. Even if you drop a few pounds, the bulk-adding embellishments will disguise it.

Q: *My husband is allergic to perfumes. For his sake, I never wear makeup or hair spray. How can I look great on my wedding day without provoking a major attack?*

Be certain that you and everyone else in your wedding party avoids the use of any products with fragrances in it. Nobody should wear perfume, and he should not come anywhere near the room where makeup or hair is being done. Use only hypoallergenic products that do not use perfumes or fixatives or ingredients that he may be allergic to. It might be helpful to him to take a medication before the wedding to prevent allergies. If he's allergic to fragrances, he could very well be allergic to the wedding flowers. If so, you should probably use silk flowers—and certainly the one he wears should not be natural.

Q: *At my wedding shower, I was mortified when my ten-year-old stepdaughter asked me why my teeth are so yellow. Is there anything I can do to brighten my smile?*

If the wedding is less than six weeks away, you can get both the top and bottom teeth lightened in an office-based bleaching session at the dentist. He applies a peroxide-based bleaching gel to the tooth surface and aims an energizing light source at your mouth to promote chemical activity. At the end of an hour, the teeth are rinsed off and the change is remarkable.

For her second
marriage,
*Audrey Hepburn wore
an archetypal 1960s
minidress in white wool.
Instead of wearing a hat
or headpiece, she covered
her long dark hair with
another symbol of the
1960s, a short kerchief.
The look was fashionably
youthful yet elegant
enough for a daytime
wedding.*

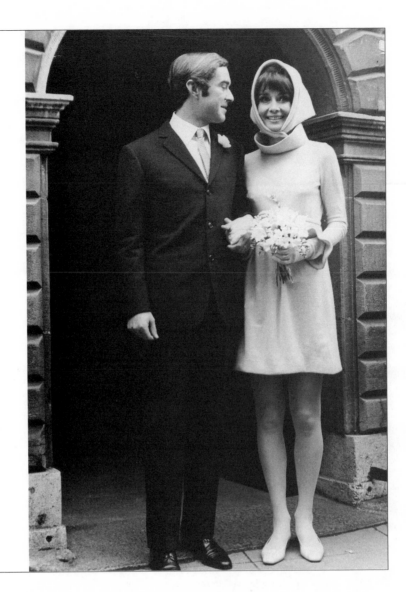

**Q. I always wanted a full, filmy wedding gown, but we've decided to have a
small, intimate wedding. Can I still wear the gown of my dreams?**

A full-skirted floor-length white gown would be a bit much for an informal wedding, but if you choose a similar style in a midcalf or ballerina
length, you would have the same fragile romantic feeling in a slightly
shorter gown. To balance the shorter length, consider wearing just a headpiece without a veil.

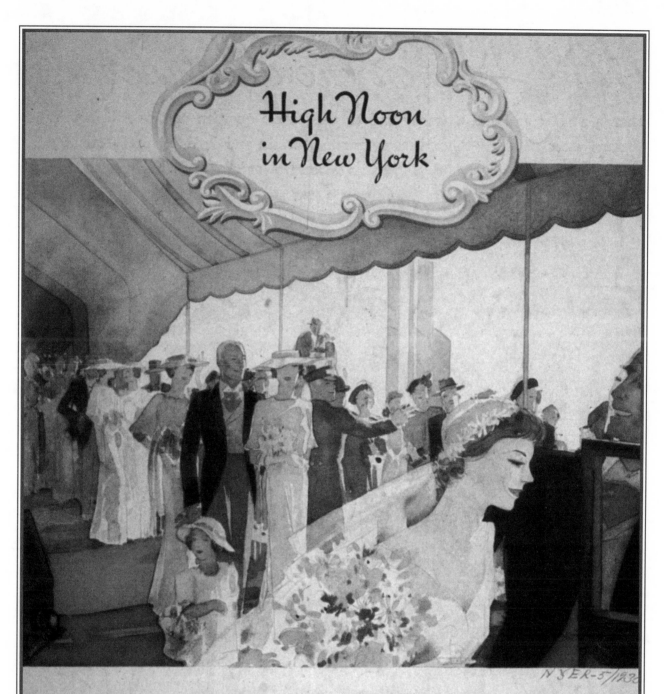

High Noon in New York

A little wistfully, perhaps, visitors witness the beauty at brilliant New York society events. To them it is a mystery how faces keep young in a city so relentlessly busy, so eternally gay. "Why, mothers here look as young as their daughters!" they exclaim.

Yet, if many of these envied matrons should tell their secret, it would be this . . . society days begin long before the clock strikes twelve, at Dorothy Gray's Fifth Avenue Salon.

To this charming salon, New York's smartest women come for rest and for Dorothy Gray's famous Salon Facial.

Skilled hands pat in softening emollients , . . pat out lines and wrinkles. And then returns a glowing freshness that triumphantly faces the brightest noon-day sun.

Do you know that you can give yourself at home the Dorothy Gray "1-2-3 Salon Facial"? Achieve the same radiant youthfulness these lovely women have? Only three simple steps:

1. Cleanse deeply, thoroughly, every night and morning, with Dorothy Gray Cream 683 . . . that fluffy cream, containing pure vegetable oils, that softens dry skin while it cleanses, $1. (If your skin is normal or oily, use Dorothy Gray Cleansing Cream, $1.)

Special Dry Skin Mixture, $2.25, $4.50. (your skin is normal or oily, use Dorothy Gr Suppling Cream, $1, $1.75, $2.75.)

3. Stimulate, after each morning cleansin with Dorothy Gray Orange Flower Sk Lotion, $.85, $1.75. (For coarse pores oily skin, use Dorothy Gray Texture Loti $1, $2.)

You will find these preparations at leadi cosmetic counters. Ask, also, for the fr booklet, "Your Lovely Skin."

© 1935, Dorothy G

Dorothy Gray

Salons at 683 Fifth Ave., New York

CHAPTER TEN

Bridal Beauty Calendar

SIX MONTHS BEFORE WEDDING

* ★ Shop for dress.
* ★ If interested in laser treatment, start to explore options.
* ★ Start growing hair.
* ★ Schedule dental assessment.
* ★ Schedule dental cleaning and polishing.
* ★ Explore hair coloring options.
* ★ Begin diet and exercise program.
* ★ Start at-home acne skin care.

FIVE MONTHS BEFORE WEDDING

* ★ Buy dress.
* ★ Start weekly facials.
* ★ Research hairstyles.
* ★ Go to cosmetic counters for makeup advice.
* ★ Interview stylists for makeup.
* ★ Begin monthly intensive hair conditioning.
* ★ Continue diet and exercise program.
* ★ If interested, schedule consultation with plastic surgeon for treatment of undereye bags.
* ★ If acne persists, schedule appointment with dermatologist.

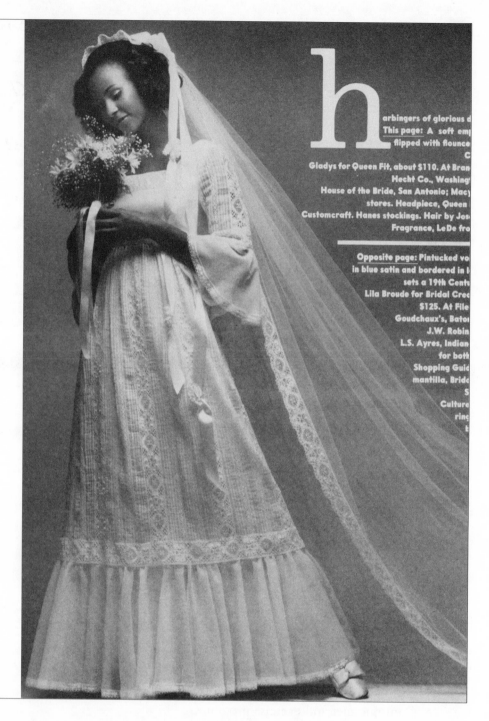

CLOSE-UP:

The 1970s Bride
....

The 1970s bride was inspired by natural shapes, fabrics, and colors. Wedding dresses were often made of cotton rather than silk and designed with a high empire waist and long, full sleeves. Hair was worn down under a small headpiece and full veil. Makeup looked very natural, even if it took many products and hours to achieve the effect. It was a democratic look worn with equal enthusiasm by society brides, rebellious college students, and small-town belles.

arbingers of glorious d
This page: A soft emp
flipped with flounce
C
Gladys for Queen Fit, about $110. At Bran
Hecht Co., Washing
House of the Bride, San Antonio; Macy
stores. Headpiece, Queen
Customcraft. Hanes stockings. Hair by Jos
Fragrance, LeDe fro

Opposite page: Pintucked vo
in blue satin and bordered in l
sets a 19th Cent
Lila Broude for Bridal Crea
$125. At File
Goudchaux's, Bato
J.W. Robin
L.S. Ayres, Indian
for both
Shopping Guid
mantilla, Brid
S
Culture
rin

Deborah

Chase

174

....
FOUR MONTHS BEFORE WEDDING
....

- ★ Start to look for headpiece.
- ★ Continue facials.
- ★ Begin intensive nail care.
- ★ Work with stylists to finalize hairstyle.
- ★ Try out different makeup styles.
- ★ Experiment with different hair-coloring techniques.

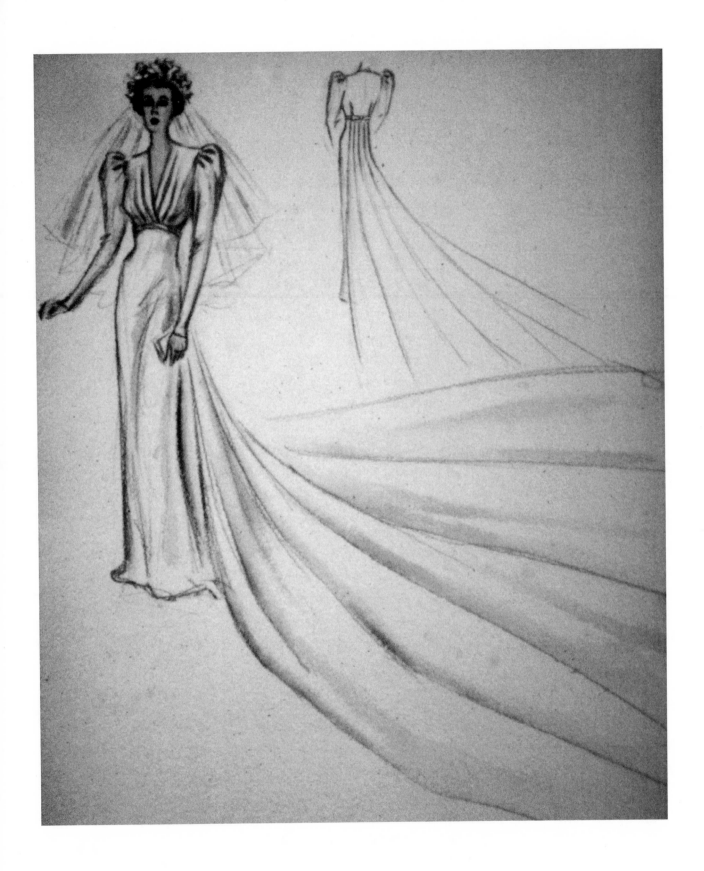

THREE MONTHS BEFORE WEDDING

* ★ Continue deep hair conditioning.
* ★ Start at-home dental bleaching.
* ★ If interested, schedule appointment for dental laminates.
* ★ Continue nail care.
* ★ Continue diet and exercise program.
* ★ Do complete hairstyle rehearsal with headpiece.
* ★ Do complete makeup rehearsal for the entire bridal party.

TWO MONTHS BEFORE WEDDING

* ★ If using professional makeup and hair stylists, make appointments for bride and bridal party.
* ★ Take first fitting of dress.
* ★ Continue facials; start glycolic peels.
* ★ Continue nail care.
* ★ Finish at home dental bleaching.
* ★ Continue diet and exercise program.
* ★ If interested, schedule laser hair removal.

ONE MONTH BEFORE WEDDING

* ★ Continue facials.
* ★ If interested, schedule in-office dental bleaching.
* ★ Have paraffin nail treatment.
* ★ If interested, schedule appointment to bond teeth.
* ★ Check wedding-day beauty supplies for self and bridal party.
* ★ Have final fitting of dress.

TWO WEEKS BEFORE WEDDING

* ★ Apply full set of fake nails, if necessary.
* ★ Schedule last facial.
* ★ Select wedding nail polish.
* ★ Continue deep hair conditioning.
* ★ Schedule last perm, if necessary.
* ★ Reconfirm time and place with hairstylist and/or makeup artist.

ONE WEEK BEFORE WEDDING

* ★ Schedule last haircut.
* ★ Wax legs, brows, and bikini line.
* ★ Schedule complete pedicure at end of week.
* ★ Apply nail tips if there is breakage.
* ★ Schedule last hair coloring.
* ★ Check wedding supply boxes.

DAY BEFORE WEDDING

* ★ Wash and condition hair.
* ★ Use mild facial sauna rather than doing a complete facial.
* ★ Do complete manicure.
* ★ Set aside two hours of quiet time to relax.

WEDDING DAY

* ★ If you are wearing an up-do, do not shampoo hair.
* ★ Schedule makeup and hair styling to begin three hours before the ceremony.
* ★ Lay out all beauty supplies where they are accessible.

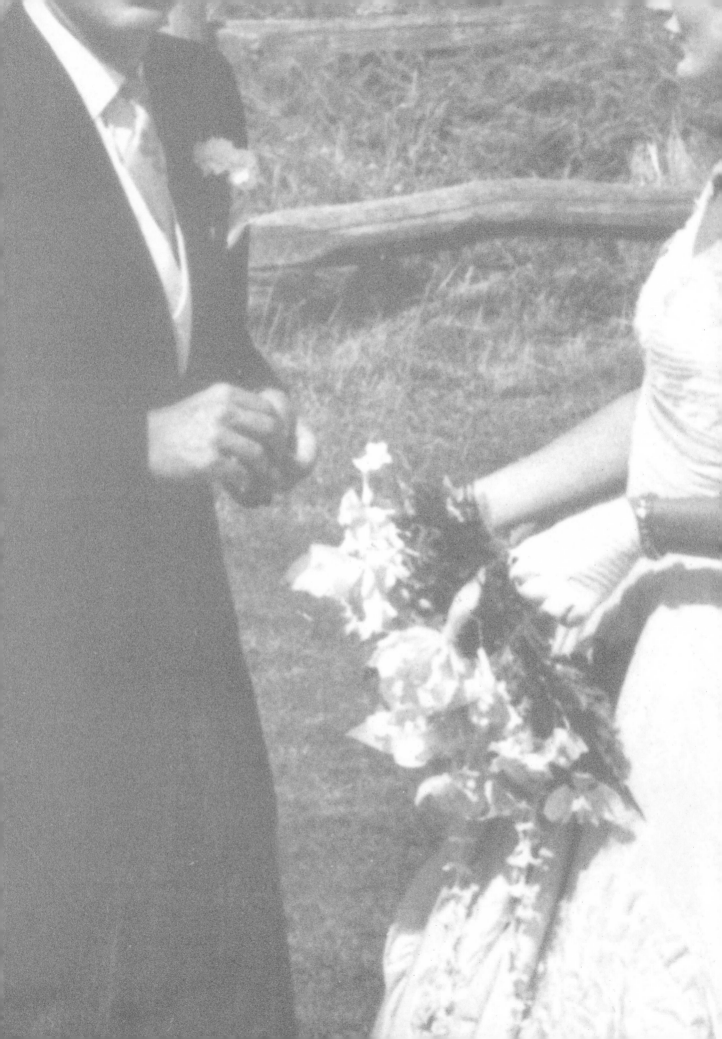

Illustration Credits